BIOETHICS

A REFORMED LOOK AT
LIFE AND DEATH CHOICES

RUTH E. GROENHOUT

FAITH
ALIVE®
Christian Resources

Grand Rapids, Michigan

Bioethics: A Reformed Look at Life and Death Choices, © 2009 by Faith Alive Christian Resources, 2850 Kalamazoo Ave. SE, Grand Rapids, MI 49560. All rights reserved. With the exception of brief excerpts for review purposes, no part of this book may be reproduced in any manner whatsoever without written permission from the publisher. Printed in the United States of America.

We welcome your comments. Call us at 1-800-333-8300, or e-mail us at editors@faithaliveresources.org.

Library of Congress Cataloging-in-Publication Data
Groenhout, Ruth E., 1962-
Bioethics: a reformed look at life and death choices / Ruth Groenhout.
    p. cm.
Includes bibliographical references.
ISBN 978-1-59255-263-4 (alk. paper)
1. Medical ethics—Religious aspects—Christianity. 2. Bioethics—Religious aspects—Christianity. 3. Christian ethics. I. Title.
R725.56.G76 2009
174'.957—dc22

                                                                2008040016

10 9 8 7 6 5 4 3 2 1

Contents

INTRODUCTION

This book offers a basic overview of some central issues in bioethics from a Christian perspective. Since the early years of the church, Christians have seen it as their duty to help provide care for the sick and dying—a mission that continues to this day. But in today's world we face questions Christians in the past never had to consider:

▸ Is it right or wrong to remove life support from a person in a persistent vegetative state?
▸ What about sperm donation or buying someone else's eggs? May we use these technologies to help infertile couples have a baby?

We worry about how Christians should respond to the fact that many Americans don't have access to health care because they're members of the "working poor"—their jobs don't provide health insurance but they make too much money to be eligible for health care through Medicaid. And we wonder about our responsibility to the poor outside our country: is it our job, as Christians, to worry about other countries' health care problems?

For most of the history of the church, these issues were not matters of concern—for the simple reason that all of them are caused by changes in technology and social structures. For instance, today we can keep people alive far past the point where their hearts and lungs would have stopped beating and breathing in earlier days. But because we can, should we? Must we? We can manipulate many individual parts of the reproductive process. But is that a good thing to do? We live in a world where health care has become very expensive and very effective at the same time. But the better it gets, the less affordable it becomes for the world's poor.

As Christians we want our thinking to be guided by Scripture and by the church community, but these aren't the sorts of questions for which we can easily find answers in Scripture. Solomon's wisdom can help us with many issues in human life, but it doesn't directly address questions about the genetic testing of embryos or about the best response to the spread of drug-resistant tuberculosis. And while the thinkers of the Christian church offer centuries of wisdom, even the best offer little direct guidance on whether we in the developed world have a moral duty to provide generic versions of antiretroviral drugs (the best preventative for

HIV/AIDS infection available) to pregnant women in third world countries to prevent transmission of the virus to babies.

For many of us, our first real confrontation with bioethics issues may be at the bedside of a dying parent when we face questions about the removal of a ventilator. That's probably a time in our life when we won't be thinking too clearly! We'll be better equipped to think through some of the difficult questions raised by contemporary health care if we consider their complexity *before* we have to deal with them concretely and personally. We'll also think more clearly about the broader issues of just access to health care and how it should be distributed if we consider the wide variety of issues involved in answering such questions.

> "If our own conversations with the families of the sick and dying are at all representative, what many people want when sickness threatens or death is at hand is a way to make sense of what is happening, or some reassurance that God will make it all come out right in the end. A conversation deserving of a lifetime of action and contemplation must necessarily be condensed into a few minutes, hours, or, at most, days."
>
> —Joel Shuman and Brian Volck, *Reclaiming the Body*

This book is designed to help the reader begin that thinking process. It doesn't offer complete coverage of every possible bioethical issue, nor does it try to describe every possible position on these issues. The aim of this book is to cover a representative range of issues, from intensely personal issues to global, policy-level concerns, and to do so from a Christian perspective shaped by faith, by the church over the past centuries, and by ongoing debate among critically engaged Christians who work on bioethics.

In the first chapter we'll look at some of the features of a Christian approach to bioethics and compare that approach to the standard model of bioethics in contemporary health care—the Principles Model. We'll note in what way the two approaches are compatible as well as how they offer different ways of thinking about bioethics. Subsequent chapters discuss specific issues—from end of life cases to ones at the beginning such as abortion and assisted reproduction; from questions about access to health care in the United States to questions about global access to health care. We'll also consider some structural questions about the focus and direction of health care. We'll be looking at both chronic diseases and conditions that require emergency treatment and considering the complex questions about how we as a society should respond to both of these.

This book won't answer all your questions about health care—in fact, it may leave you with more questions than when you started! What it will do is help you to recognize what sorts of ethical issues arise in health care, why they arise, and what sorts of responses are available. Because we live in a complex world, the problems of bioethics don't have easy answers. Every solution to a single problem seems to generate several other difficulties! But Scripture calls us to be wise. In the area of bioethics, a large part of wisdom is recognizing the complexities of our world so that we don't offer simplistic answers to complicated questions. It's our hope that this book will generate the kind of discussion that leads to the beginning of wisdom about bioethics.

CHAPTER 1

CHRISTIANS, HEALTH CARE, AND BASIC MORAL REASONING

Lila Nichols sits opposite her pastor, Charles Kim. They're in his office, a grey Michigan sky framed in the window. "Pancreatic cancer has a really low long-term survival rate," she says. "The doctors are giving me less than six months to live. I'm thinking about contacting hospice and just having low-level chemotherapy to slow the progress of the cancer. I want to skip the aggressive treatment that one of my doctors is recommending. But my friend Martha keeps telling me that I'm giving up. She says that's the same thing as suicide. What do you think?"

Pastor Kim shakes his head. "I'm so sorry to hear this, Lila. I don't think hospice is the same thing as suicide, but I'd like to talk about it with you. How can the church be there for you right now?"

"Oh, I don't want the church to know," she says emphatically. "I'll tell a few close friends, but I don't want people in church talking about me. In fact, I thought about not coming anymore. I don't want people to see me getting worse, and I don't want to be a bother. So I really don't want you to tell anyone. Like I said, I just wanted to see if you think hospice is the same as suicide. And please don't get any ideas about having people pray for me. I don't need any of that right now."

"If you don't want people to come and pray for you, I'll respect your wishes," says Pastor Kim. "But I do think you need to rethink the plan to keep this private. This is the sort of thing that should be shared with the church, and I think you'll find that you get a lot of support and love when you do."

♦ ♦ ♦ ♦ ♦ ♦ ♦

In this chapter we'll look at a biblical framework for thinking about bioethical decisions, beginning with the centrality of healing as a sign of God's kingdom in the world. Scripture is full of stories of healing: from the healing miracles so central to Jesus' ministry, to Elisha's healing of his patron's son, to the use of healing as a description of God's love in the prophets.

Clearly spiritual health is important, but we should never lose sight of the fact that Scripture draws close connections between our physical and spiritual health. The brokenness of the fall leads to disease and death, and the redemption achieved through Jesus' death brings both spiritual and physical healing—and ultimately, the overcoming of death altogether. Given that emphasis, it makes sense to ask how Christians should approach issues of health and sickness, of medicine and faith healing, and of new technologies and the timeless recognition that we humans do get sick and die.

THE CHURCH AS COMMUNITY

One of the most important features of our lives as Christians is the fact that we don't make life and death decisions all by ourselves. We are connected to God and to each other. That's why Christian thinking about medicine and bioethics differs from the standard models of bioethics taught in medical schools across the country. Those models emphasize individual autonomy and protecting the patient's right to make decisions—both very important issues. But their focus is on people as isolated individuals, not as members of a community.

Two sets of considerations, then, structure our thought as Christians about controversial and difficult issues in bioethics. The first deals with how we make decisions as members of the body of Christ. How does that help shape the decisions we make and the way we make them?

The second relates to the way the church as a whole should respond to bioethical issues. What we choose to do and say as the body of Christ provides an image of God to the world. How can we faithfully reflect who God is to those around us? Can our response to bioethical issues make visible the good news of God's love and redemption? These questions need to shape our reasoning about bioethics so that our decisions and actions reflect Christ in our lives.

Shaped by these two sets of considerations, the central focus of this book is not so much on individual decision-making in standard bioethics mode, but rather on how the Christian community can respond faithfully to the health care issues and needs around us.

THE STORIES OF SCRIPTURE SHAPE OUR LIVES

One of the first things we need to recognize is that a community's identity is shaped by stories. This is obviously true for the church—a community that historically has found its identity in the stories of Scripture. The stories of Scripture tell us who we are and where we come from. They tell us about the goals of our actions and our lives. For Christians, the most important story has three parts: the story of God's creation of the world; the human fall from a right relationship with God into one marked by conflict, separation, and sin; and God's redemption of right relationships through the life, death, and resurrection of Jesus. It's the story of a future we look forward to—a world made whole again by God's grace.

> "These stories are not situated within the world: instead, for the Christian, the world is situated within these stories."
>
> —John Milbank (Quoted in Joel Shuman, *Heal Thyself*)

This overarching structure allows us to see that the world God created is good and that it was made for a purpose—for God's enjoyment and for our flourishing. In the health care context, we see this basic goodness of creation in any number of ways:

- in the almost miraculous way bodies can heal themselves, given half a chance
- in the way humans develop from embryos into babies, then into adults who grow and flourish physically and emotionally
- in the ways people reach out to each other to help, to care, and to express love
- in the wonderful capacity medicine has to heal and to save lives that would otherwise be lost

People who work in the field of health care see all sorts of wonderful structures and events that we can celebrate as the good gifts of God.

But life is not all good. We live in a world that is full of broken relationships, sinful choices, tragic illnesses, and death. This too is part of the story Scripture tells. Things are not all right with the world, and we can see this in the context of medicine:

- People get sick and sometimes there's no cure.
- People hurt each other deliberately and by negligence; health care workers have to care for the broken bodies and suffering minds of those damaged by others.

- People die despite our best efforts; in some really hard cases people die *because* of what health care workers have done to them.
- Even when medicine can offer a cure, it doesn't always restore a person to complete health. Medicine that slows the progress of a disease can have side effects that make a person miserable. Surgery to correct one condition can generate other problems that can't be fixed.

Christians experience both aspects of the world: its basic goodness and its corruption by sin. But we aren't just passive bystanders. God created us to be active participants in the world, engaging in the unfolding story that God is writing. Our job is to live in ways that reflect our hope in the good future God is bringing about. This gives us a context for making sense of what happens to us and for figuring out how to live as the body of Christ in the world.

> "Reading Scripture trains us to see the religious significance of events, to read the signs of the times in the things that are happening about us, and to locate events and circumstances—as well as our selves—in a story of God's power and grace."
>
> —Allen Verhey, *Reading the Bible in the Strange World of Medicine*

Christian thinkers and writers, including ethicist Allen Verhey, have argued that one of our central tasks as the body of Christ is to become the sort of people and the sort of community that represent God to the world. The good news of God's love needs to be visible in us. That's much easier said than done: it isn't hard to *talk* about being a loving community, but anyone who's been a member of a church for very long knows that actually *doing* it can seem pretty much impossible on the bad days, and tough even on good ones.

Developing the character traits we need to live together as a loving community doesn't happen overnight. If I want to be a gentle, generous, honest person, I have to spend years practicing those characteristics until they become so ingrained in me that it would be difficult to act dishonestly or selfishly. That takes hard work and extensive practice! And few of us have the discipline on our own to really work at it. (After all, working on character fitness is a good deal harder than working on physical fitness, and most of us can't even do the latter!) That's where community comes in. The church provides us with a group of people working on the same issues. Together we can schedule times to do volunteer work and meet together to talk about issues we're struggling with. Together we can find ways to practice the virtues we should exhibit to the world.

We recognize a person's character by her or his actions, but also by how that person resolves problems. Communities are the same. We recognize the character of a community by how it identifies, speaks to, and resolves problems. A church that says it follows Jesus but resorts to character attacks and underhanded dealings when confronted with conflict reflects badly on Jesus' name. Our actions as the body of Christ leave a stronger impression in the world than the words we use or the sermons we preach.

When the church community embodies God's love and grace to its members, it has the potential to be a powerful force in society. In the context of bioethics, for example, a church community that reaches out to its members struggling with chronic illness, supports them, loves them, and keeps them enfolded in the community is a church that can speak credibly to the world about the needs of those who deal with chronic illness.

SOCIETAL STRUCTURES AND REDEMPTION

Psychologist Mary Stewart Van Leeuwen notes that Scripture uses the language of "principalities and powers" when speaking about the social structures of human life. The "powers" are social forces that shape and even determine the ways we can act in the world. They are so big and so entrenched that no single individual can simply decide to set them aside. We live in a world structured by a global economic system, for example, and whether we like it or not, that fact shapes our lives and our options. Other powers that shape us include family structures, economic structures, political structures, education systems, and (most centrally for our purposes) medicine.

Sometimes these powers take on a life of their own, like Frankenstein's monster. When they claim to determine the whole meaning of human life, they become idols—they stand in the place of God. Medicine, for example, is a powerful and complex social structure. People turn to medicine for health, safety, and meaning in an uncertain world.

- For those who are sick and dying, medicine offers healing and comfort.
- For those who are dissatisfied with their lives, medicine offers diets and cosmetic surgery.

- For those who feel their lives have no meaning, medicine offers antidepressants and mood enhancers.
- These can all be good things. But none of them are "the pearl of great price" Jesus refers to in Matthew 13:46 (KJV), and if we start thinking they are, we're in trouble.

> "The alternative to the idolatry that is bondage to the powers is the proper worship of God. By *worship* we mean . . . the entire orientation of lives that have been shaped by the repeated retelling and reenactment of the Christian story on Sunday mornings."
>
> —Joel Shuman and Brian Volck, *Reclaiming the Body*

In the abstract, of course, it is relatively easy to see that medicine should not be the central focus of our lives. But in the midst of a medical crisis—when our child is diagnosed with cancer or when we're struggling with infertility—it can become very easy to find all our hopes and dreams resting on the outcome of the next diagnostic test or the latest technological procedure. When this happens, not only are we placing our hope in the wrong place, we are placing it in a system that cannot hope to truly satisfy. Medicine is a good thing, but it cannot stave off death forever or repair broken lives. And like other idols, it will betray us.

Many of us, in fact, have experienced this sense of betrayal to some degree. A hip replacement, for example, may offer the hope of new life and perfect function. But though we can expect a good deal of improvement after a hip replacement, we are unlikely to ever feel "new" again. And no matter how much we turn to medicine for relief of the "symptoms" of aging by undergoing plastic surgery, vitamin therapy, Botox injections, or hormone replacement, our bodies continue to age.

It's not hard to see that medicine is a power in our lives—a force that appears to offer meaning, wholeness, and healing to us in almost magical ways. So we react with anger and bitterness when medicine turns out to be a fallible, human practice. After all, the mistakes and limitations of medicine are lived out in our very flesh. When my hip replacement doesn't work well, it's *my* body that aches every day. When a surgeon makes a mistake, *I'm* the one forced to wear a colostomy bag.

Many of the lawsuits brought against doctors are filed by those who feel betrayed. These people thought medicine could solve their problems, but it didn't. No one wants to be in that small percentage of people who don't survive general anesthesia, but the reality is that there is a risk, and some people will die. We have an image of medicine as all-powerful, offering solutions for the problems that we worry about. The suspicion and hatred people sometimes feel toward doctors and medicine as a whole is the dark side of the idolatry of medicine.

Christians have an alternative view of the power of medicine. We can appreciate its tremendous power and its resources for good. But we know that medicine is not a god who will save us if we sacrifice sufficient money and resources in its name. And if we pursue immortality through medicine, we will fail at the tasks that we should be pursuing: living the lives God has called us to and serving the needs of others. Ultimately we recognize that medicine is an important part of human life, one that should be situated within God's larger plan as one important good among many—never the ultimate good.

THE LANGUAGE OF BIOETHICS: PRINCIPLES-BASED REASONING

So far we've talked about how the Christian community might understand its own relationship to the practices of modern medicine. But when people find themselves dealing with the health care system, it isn't enough to be able to frame medicine within a Christian worldview. We also need to be able to translate our values and beliefs into language that makes sense to doctors, nurses, and sometimes administrators who may not have much concern for or understanding of Christian perspectives.

Contemporary bioethics is fundamentally shaped by *principles-based reasoning*, a method developed by James Childress and Tom Beauchamp in their book, *Principles of Biomedical Ethics*. The four principles they developed offer a common language for medical professionals and others to talk about ethics and resolve conflicts:

- ▶ autonomy (respect the patient's right to make decisions)
- ▶ beneficence (help others)
- ▶ nonmaleficence (do no harm)
- ▶ justice (make sure burdens and benefits are fairly distributed)

Autonomy refers to the patient's right to make decisions about her or his own care. It includes the right to be informed about available treatments, the nature of any proposed interventions, and the side effects and probable outcomes of those interventions.

Beneficence identifies the central medical goal of helping others. *Nonmaleficence* refers to the moral duty to refrain from doing harm.

Sometimes it is hard to distinguish between benefiting others and refraining from harm, but they do differ. Doctors may focus so single-mindedly on trying to cure a patient, for example, that they lose sight of the harm their techniques may cause. Separating beneficence and nonmaleficence reminds us to balance trying to help and avoiding harm.

Finally, the principle of *justice* reminds us that health care must be available to those who need it, whether in individual cases, as when many people want access to a particularly scarce resource (as often happens in organ donation) or on a broader scale, such as the huge number of people without access to basic health care in some countries, including the United States.

Being able to refer to these principles provides a helpful context for discussing health care among people who may have lots of different ideas about ethics and moral responsibilities. Because they work pretty well in that capacity, they've become standard in many discussions of bioethics.

But as is always the case, the more general our principles are, the harder it is to apply them in specific situations. For example, when debating whether or not it is acceptable to remove a ventilator from someone in a persistent vegetative state, one person may say that it would be a benefit to keep the patient breathing (a fairly obvious benefit!); another may argue that extending the dying process over a long period of time actually harms the patient. There's no easy way to resolve such conflict if the principles themselves are our only resource.

"A persistent vegetative state, which sometimes follows a coma, refers to a condition in which individuals have lost cognitive neurological function and awareness of the environment but retain noncognitive function and a preserved sleep-wake cycle.

"It is sometimes described as when a person is technically alive, but his/her brain is dead. However, that description is not completely accurate. In persistent vegetative state, the individual loses the higher cerebral powers of the brain, but the functions of the brainstem, such as respiration (breathing) and circulation, remain relatively intact. Spontaneous movements may occur and the eyes may open in response to external stimuli, but the patient does not speak or obey commands. Patients in a vegetative state may appear somewhat normal. They may occasionally grimace, cry, or laugh."

—Healthlink, Medical College of Wisconsin

A Christian perspective offers other resources to draw from. Situating the bioethical principles we've described within the context of Scripture and the Christian tradition gives us a rich source of material for thinking about bioethics.

1. Autonomy

Let's start with the principle of autonomy, which reminds us that the related concepts of freedom and responsibility are crucial components of human life. Because I can choose from a variety of options, I am also responsible for what I choose. If I have no options or am unable to choose, I can't (realistically) be held responsible for what happens.

Our culture tends to equate diminished health and vigor with diminished humanity. Friends of mine who use wheelchairs, for example, recount stories of people looking past them as if they can't speak. And the elderly are routinely treated as incompetent or invisible. As Christians who recognize the image of God in all people, we need to counter this cultural bias by respecting the autonomy of everyone, healthy or sick, old or young, vulnerable or strong. But as Allen Verhey reminds us, autonomy doesn't mean leaving people alone to make whatever decision they want. Christians know that true autonomy is best exercised in community, in conversation with those who know and love us best.

2. Beneficence

The second principle reminds us that we have a duty to help others. Both the Old and New Testaments are so full of God's commands to feed the hungry and care for the widowed, the orphaned, and the foreigner that it is impossible not to see connections between beneficence and a Christian worldview.

The Christian call to protect and help the weak and vulnerable in society forms an important background to medical history. The early church created communities devoted to the care of the sick and the elderly. Hospitals were originally shelters created for the sick and weary on pilgrimages. The church community frequently made houses of refuge and care for the sick a central part of their ministry; even today the names of many hospitals across North America point to their historical connection to one or another Christian community.

This historical perspective suggests one significant difference from the general principle of beneficence. While beneficence may sometimes be a matter of one individual helping another (as in the parable of the Good Samaritan), the church historically has seen this as a collective duty. The needs of the poor and vulnerable are likely to require structural solutions: institutions, funding, specialized training, and long-term commitments. As Christians we are called to help in ways that make a real difference.

From a Christian perspective, the principle of beneficence also needs to address the tendency to focus only on physical life and health. As important as both of these are, they need to be set within the broader context of the spiritual and social aspects of human life. A person is never merely a body to be fixed and sent on its way but is rather someone who lives in relation to God and to others.

3. Nonmaleficence

The third principle cautions us to avoid as much as possible the harm that can be caused by the practice of medicine. Again, Christians have a particular perspective on this principle. Most folks recognize that when medicine causes more physical problems than it solves it is bad medicine. But Christians are also aware, as we noted earlier, of the temptation to put our whole trust and faith in the practice of medicine, to think that doctors can fix all that is broken in our lives.

4. Justice

This final principle naturally resonates with Christians. Scripture is full of commands to do justice, especially when those who have power use their position to manipulate or exploit those who are weaker. In the field of health care, this sort of exploitation can take any number of forms. Poorer countries, for example, have recently struggled with forced "donations" of kidneys. These organs are sold to wealthy Westerners willing to pay a premium price for an organ that is not readily available in North America or Europe. Other injustices are more systemic: because of the huge disparities in wealth between poor nations and wealthier ones, only the wealthy have access to premium health care, while the poorest have minimal or no health care. Christians bring to their discussion about justice the conviction that all humans have value, not just those who are wealthy.

When we as Christians find ourselves maneuvering through the health care system, the four principles we've discussed give us a language that caregivers will understand. But we need to flesh out these basic ideas with the broader perspective our faith makes available.

CONCLUSION

Christians approach bioethics from a number of different viewpoints. One of the things this book aims to do is look at how different Christians have approached various bioethical issues, what conclusions they have reached, and why. We will not offer quick or simplistic solutions—after all, most bioethical issues are debated precisely because they are complicated and difficult and because they represent areas where there are deep conflicts of interest between individuals or groups. Responsible Christian freedom requires us to think for ourselves when discussing the issues we'll cover in this book.

At the same time, Christians need to recognize God's guidance as we think through difficult issues. Our stories are situated in the context of Scripture. As children of God, we are called to be light and salt to the world. We're called to live out God's love and compassion for other people and the rest of creation. Further, we don't make decisions as isolated individuals. We live as members of God's family, a community into which we have been baptized. Our church community is both immediate (the folks we see in church) and very far away (Christians living on the other side of the world, often in very difficult situations). The church is a community with a long history and with enormous wisdom accumulated through ages of thinking about what it means to be a follower of Christ.

> "To speak properly of health we need to describe the place where the personal and the communal intersect. The freedom that is health cannot be found in solitude: it is a freedom found when we humans learn to cooperate . . . to reach a common goal."
>
> —Alastair V. Campbell, *Health as Liberation*

In our discussion about bioethics we'll try to listen carefully to what other Christians say and to what modern medicine can tell us. We'll also think for ourselves. We'll consider alternative viewpoints and the reasons that Christians might disagree about some of these issues. Finally, we'll try to adopt an attitude of gentleness, humility, and respect for those who may not agree with us. Scripture commands us to seek wisdom; it also reminds us that for now we see only through a glass darkly. We'll try to remember that tension as we think about the various bioethical issues of our day.

Questions for Reflection and Discussion

1. How would you counsel Lila if you were Pastor Kim in the scenario at the beginning of the chapter? What other issues, if any, should be explored?

2. Review and evaluate the four principles widely used in discussing bio-ethics. How does our membership in the family of God add to or shape the discussion?

3. This chapter uses the language of "principalities and powers" to talk about social structures such as health care. How does the power of medicine and health care tempt us to idolatry? How can a Christian perspective help us to see medicine in its proper place?

4. Healing is central to the ways Scripture portrays the kingdom of God. How can churches build a concern for healing into their ministries?

For Further Reading

Doornbos, Mary Molewyk, Ruth E. Groenhout, and Kendra G. Hotz. *Transforming Care: A Christian Vision of Nursing Practice.* Grand Rapids, Mich.: Eerdmans, 2005.

Mohrmann, Margaret E., M.D. *Medicine as Ministry: Reflections on Suffering, Ethics, and Hope.* Cleveland: The Pilgrim Press, 1995

Shuman, Joel and Brian Volck, M.D. *Reclaiming the Body: Christians and the Faithful Use of Modern Medicine.* Grand Rapids, Mich.: Brazos Press, 2006.

Verhey, Allen. *Reading the Bible in the Strange World of Medicine.* Grand Rapids, Mich.: Eerdmans, 2003.

CHAPTER 2

WHEN LIFE ENDS

D r. Cheng is presenting a case to the ethics committee of Lutheran General Hospital. "Today we're asked to think about another end of life case. The patient, a seventy-one-year-old man, was admitted to Emergency last night, complaining of dizziness and chest pain. He has a history of diabetes and kidney failure and has been undergoing dialysis, but this time the chest pains are from an MI. We did what we could for him last night—today he's on a ventilator and not conscious."

Ken, a member of the committee, stops her. "What's an MI? I'm a pastor, not a medical person."

"Myocardial infarction. Heart attack. This guy has arteriosclerosis, so his heart muscle can't get the oxygen it needs. He also has a pacemaker, but it's failing because of a bacterial infection. Normally we'd replace the pacemaker, but with all the other conditions—kidneys, diabetes, infection—it's unlikely he'd survive the surgery, and the infection is likely to reoccur."

"So what's the ethical issue?" asks Janice, a nurse.

"The family's demanding we do everything," Dr. Cheng says, shaking her head. "The only family is a nephew. He says he wants everything possible done to keep his uncle alive—that's what his uncle would have wanted. The social worker thinks he's trying to make up for guilt feelings by demanding treatment."

"Insurance?" asks Jeremy, the hospital attorney.

"Nope, Medicaid," responds Dr. Cheng. "So we're already looking at a fairly substantial amount of care that won't be paid for. But the real question is, what does it mean for us to do everything? Should we even tell the nephew that surgery to replace the pacemaker is an option? None of the surgeons want to do it because it doesn't look like the patient can survive the surgery, but without the pacemaker he's going to die. The nephew doesn't want a DNR, so it looks as though we're also stuck doing resuscitation."

Looking at Ken, she explains, "DNR means 'do not resuscitate.' It means we don't have to try to restore breathing or heart function if his heart stops again. If we try to resuscitate this poor guy, we'll be putting him through absolute misery—shoving tubes down his throat, shocking him. I've seen ribs broken during chest compressions . . . and for what? So we can do it all over ten minutes later when he codes again? He's dying, for pete's sake. I know his nephew thinks he's doing the right thing, but if he loved his uncle, he'd let him die peacefully."

◆ ◆ ◆ ◆ ◆ ◆ ◆

Cases like this make up almost half of the decisions facing hospital ethics committees. Family members, in shock when their loved ones are suddenly facing death, want to hold off death by any means. Physicians and nurses are horrified at the thought of having to force all sorts of needless and possibly painful treatment on a dying patient. And the patients—either because they're heavily sedated or unconscious or unable to think clearly—often have nothing to say.

As Christians we want to approach medical care at the end of life in ways that embody our faith and our commitment to a God of life. But the truth is that Christians disagree about what that means.

A BRIEF HISTORY OF HEALTH CARE

The way we die has undergone enormous changes in the past century. A hundred years ago, only poor people routinely died in hospitals, which were designed to provide comfort and care for the poor and indigent. Patients shared a large ward with very little privacy, and family members were kept strictly away—except for the two or three visiting hours allowed per week. Wealthy people, on the other hand, stayed home and had their doctor come to them. They were able to spend their last hours at home in the presence of family members and a doctor or perhaps a private nurse.

Over the course of the twentieth century, medicine went through radical changes. In 1900 there were no antibiotics and few treatments other than cleanliness, some basic surgeries, aspirin, and morphine. By 1950 antibiotics had become widely available (penicillin was developed in the 1940s), and doctors were performing surgeries that were far more complex (and more often successful). The medical repertoire expanded to include tools such as X-ray imaging, blood transfusions, and more effective medications. As medicine increased in complexity, hospitals began to offer more medical treatments, and by the 1970s, most births and deaths took place in a hospital setting. These days, doctors perform procedures that had not even been dreamed of in 1900. But even with all the technology and pharmaceuticals available to us today, we still die.

The advancements in health care we enjoy in the twenty-first century mean that we're faced with a whole new set of questions:

▸ Because we live in a world where we can extend life beyond its natural ending point, we need to ask whether such extensions are good or not so good.

▸ Because we live in a world where people end their lives unconscious and sedated, surrounded by technology and machines, we need to ask if there aren't better ways to die.

▸ Because we live in a world where, regardless of how much progress medicine has made, some still suffer terribly at the end of life, we need to ask, why does such suffering exist? Why does God allow it, and is it always wrong to end it by shortening life?

Let's start with a slightly less difficult question: Who should make decisions at the end of life, and what sorts of decisions should be made?

WHO MAKES DECISIONS?

Legally, the question of who makes decisions at the end of life is relatively simple. The person who is dying has the legal right to choose or to reject medical treatments so long as she or he is competent to understand the procedure and to make decisions about it. If that's not the case, in most states the right to make decisions shifts either to the next of kin (in order: spouse, parent or adult child, next closest relative) or to the person designated by a Durable Power of Attorney Form that designates another individual as a legal guardian or to a designated Health Care Representative.

A Durable Power of Attorney takes precedence over any other type of relationship. If you don't want your children making decisions for you at the end of life, make sure you fill out such a form. If you do want your children making decisions, then don't fill out such a form listing someone else as guardian, or your children will have no say in what happens. It's also possible to appoint someone as your Health Care Representative by filling out and signing the appropriate forms, authorizing this person to make health care decisions on your behalf in case you are unable to make such decisions.

But the legal question is not our central concern. Who *should* be making decisions about issues at the end of life? We live in a culture that emphasizes the individual's autonomy, but as we noted in chapter 1, Christians belong to a community. We profess that we belong to Jesus, not to ourselves.

Knowing that we belong to God allows us to relax a bit, even under the difficult circumstances of hospitalization and the need to make sudden decisions. We do not go through sickness or death alone. And because God is with us, we don't approach these trials without hope. At one level, nothing changes. We still have to make the tough decisions about when to start or stop a ventilator, for instance. But at another level we can make decisions prayerfully, in the knowledge that whether we live or die is not our own responsibility.

> **Q. What is your only comfort in life and in death?**
> **A.** That I am not my own, but belong—body and soul, in life and in death—to my faithful Savior Jesus Christ. . . .
>
> —The Heidelberg Catechism, Q&A 1

Belonging to God also means recognizing that we can make our difficult decisions in consultation with the community of Christ. If there is ever a time to call your pastor and ask for prayer and advice, this is it! If you don't feel comfortable calling your pastor or elder, or anyone else from your church community, perhaps you need to wonder whether you are going to the right church. What sorts of help can you reasonably expect from your church family?

▸ First, remember that making decisions in community does not mean turning authority over to someone else. The individual and family members are the ones designated to make decisions for a reason— they know the person best, what sorts of decisions are appropriate, and how their decisions will fit with other parts of their lives. The prayers, the presence, the emotional support of your church community won't make the pain of death go away, but they will alleviate the terrible loneliness that can otherwise accompany the end of life.

▸ Second, your church family can help you see alternatives and support you as you think through your decisions. In the health care setting it can be easy to assume automatically that the correct response to a crisis is to react aggressively with as much technology as possible. That's because hospitals are designed to deliver health care, not to help people ask whether particular aspects of health care are the best thing to pursue. We're told that if we perform this procedure, this surgery, or this intervention, there's a chance of recovery, of prolonging life, of improvement.

This is not to say that health care teams will always suggest doing everything possible in a medical crisis. As we saw in the case study that began this chapter, ethics committees frequently deal with families who want "everything to be done" for their loved one, even when caregivers believe that such efforts will be unsuccessful and will cause the patient additional misery. Informing people about all available treatments and procedures is part of the hospital's job, and in the emotional chaos and the sense of desperation we feel when our loved one is dying, we are likely to grab hold of anything that seems to offer any hope of improvement.

This is why having the church community with you when facing end-of-life decisions is so important. Other people who love you will have some distance from the situation. They may help you sort out which treatments are unlikely to offer any reasonable hope of cure or restoration. And they can support you as you make decisions, pray with you, and surround you with a sense of community.

WHAT IS END-OF-LIFE CARE?

Decisions about end-of-life care may address a variety of different issues. The most basic issue—DNR, or Do Not Resuscitate—came up in the scenario that began this chapter. Doctors and nurses are required by law to try to resuscitate patients if they stop breathing or if their heart stops beating. This makes sense, of course, since people who are in a hospital are there to be taken care of.

Resuscitation is a traumatic event. When someone stops breathing, caregivers may use a combination of techniques to try to get the person breathing again. These include pushing oxygen into the lungs through either a mask or a tracheotomy (a hole cut into the neck to allow a ventilator tube); chest compressions, in which doctors push hard on the ribs to try to get the heart to start beating again; open chest heart massage; or electric shock with a defibrillator unit to get the heart beating.

If there is a chance the patient will be revived, it makes good sense to resuscitate her or him. But when someone is extremely sick, resuscitation is unlikely to accomplish any particular positive outcome. Patients whose organ systems are failing all at once, or those who are particularly frail or elderly, are extremely unlikely to benefit. In these cases caregivers generally encourage the patient or the family to issue a Do Not Resuscitate (DNR) order on the patient's chart. This doesn't mean the hospital staff will stop caring for the person; it just means that if the patient stops breathing, the hospital staff will allow her to die peacefully. If no DNR order has been issued, the staff must attempt resuscitation.

Another decision that may arise in end-of-life care is whether to use a ventilator. A person who is very ill often needs a ventilator (or respirator— pretty much the same thing) to help with breathing. Ventilators help in two ways—they can add pressure to force air into a person's lungs, and they can deliver concentrated quantities of oxygen. This sort of help can allow the body to survive while other organ systems heal. Unfortunately many people do not want to use ventilators because they are afraid of becoming dependent—that is, being permanently hooked up to a ventilator.

It used to be the case that doctors equated taking a patient off a ventilator with causing the person's death. Many doctors were reluctant to start a patient on a ventilator, especially a frail or elderly patient, because they were afraid that once the treatment was started, it couldn't be ended. This led to a careful distinction between *withholding* treatment (not putting someone on it in the first place) and *withdrawing* treatment (taking it away once it had been started). Legally, however, (at least in the United States, Canada, and Great Britain) there is no difference between withholding and withdrawing treatment. So it makes more sense to try using a ventilator, with the option of removing it if it isn't helping.

Feeding tubes are another end-of-life concern. When people are unable to take in sufficient nourishment by mouth because of paralysis, senility, or surgery, doctors can insert a feeding tube through the nose and into the stomach or directly into the abdomen, allowing them to receive food and fluids.

These basic technologies are of enormous benefit for many people, but they have a downside as well. Because it is possible to keep people alive by using ventilators and feeding tubes, we frequently do. Whether this is always a good thing is a matter of serious debate. Many people, for example, express a deep fear of ventilator dependency: "If I'm ever in a coma I'd want people to pull the plug." Many think that extending a person's life with increasingly invasive technological interventions that don't ultimately improve the patient's life is wrong.

A GOOD DEATH?

One response to this "downside" of using technology to prolong life has been the use of technology to end life. Groups such as the Hemlock Society argue that providing the means to voluntarily end one's life should be part of contemporary health care. The term used for actively hastening the death of a terminally ill person is *euthanasia*, a word that means "good death." Some European countries have legalized euthanasia, usually by lethal injection, under fairly restricted conditions.

Proponents of euthanasia argue that allowing people who are suffering to have their lives ended quickly and compassionately is a vital part of the medical mission. Critics say medicine should never be used to actively cause a person's death. Since medicine is oriented toward life and healing, they argue, direct killing, even if done compassionately, is contrary to the basic structure of medical care. Further, any legalization of euthanasia, even under restricted circumstances, leads to a willingness to use lethal techniques in a broader range of cases: for example, from using lethal injection to end the lives of terminal patients to ending the life of newborns with severe but non-life-threatening disabilities. (This is often called the "slippery slope" argument.) Finally, critics argue, euthanasia puts the dying under terrible pressure to "get it over with." People who are dying should not have to face the psychological pressure of knowing that people are willing to kill them quickly.

There is evidence supporting the "slippery slope" concern from the Netherlands, the first country to legalize euthanasia. While the original legislation limited euthanasia to individuals who requested it, the practice has been extended to handicapped newborns, individuals in a persistent vegetative state (see p. 16), and others who are unable to make direct requests.

As originally written, the law in the Netherlands permitted euthanasia only when the following conditions are met:
- ▸ The patient is competent and initiates the request.
- ▸ The patient is experiencing unbearable suffering.
- ▸ The patient is informed about alternatives, does not suffer from depression, and expresses the request for euthanasia firmly and consistently.
- ▸ The physician must consult with another physician and submit a report to the government that documents the patient's condition and wishes.

Euthanasia is illegal in the United States and Canada, although various groups have tried to pass legislation that would allow it. In 1994, Oregon passed the Death with Dignity Act, making it legal for physicians to prescribe lethal drugs for terminally ill patients without risking criminal prosecution. However, the law does not permit physicians to *administer* a lethal injection, but only to prescribe a medicine that can cause death. As a result, this practice is called physician assisted suicide rather than euthanasia. The Oregon law has survived a variety of legal challenges from the federal government, and since 1998 a small but relatively steady number of people have used the procedure to end their lives each year.

In response to the right to die movement, many Christian groups began to recognize that different sorts of care are needed for the dying than for those who are fighting illness. Ironically, hospice care became a reality in response to euthanasia and physician assisted suicide. Hospice focuses on providing quality of life during the dying process—emphasizing pain control, minimizing technological interferences, and encouraging the dying to spend their last days with people they love.

Hospice care focuses on addressing some central goals:
- To support individuals and families coping with dying.
- To enhance quality of life through comfort care rather than treatment focused on cure.
- To aggressively treat and expertly manage all pain and physical symptoms associated with an individual's dying.
- To care for the whole person, addressing physical, emotional, psychological, spiritual, and social needs through an interdisciplinary team approach.
- To confirm the individual's and family's sense of self worth, individuality, autonomy, and security.
- To acknowledge and offer support for individuals and their family members facing the losses and grief associated with dying and the death of a loved one.
- To extend bereavement support for family members following the death of their loved one.
- To be a positive influence upon the understanding, compassionate treatment, and care of the dying and bereaved.

—Lattanzi-Licht, Mahoney, & Miller, *Hospice Choice:*
In Pursuit of a Peaceful Death

Hospice and euthanasia share some of the same values. Both emphasize the relief of suffering and focus on the patient's experience at the end of life. Both are responses to a health care system that is very good at treating conditions aggressively but not so good at stopping when the treatment is no longer helping. But there is a fundamental difference in perspective between the two. Hospice recognizes that death is approaching and uses medical treatment to make the patient's last days as good as possible. In contrast, euthanasia embraces death as an end to suffering.

Many Christian thinkers reject euthanasia. Allen Verhey, for example, argues that we as Christians are to position ourselves on the side of life, not death. But, he continues, we can't stop there. If we simply say that suicide is not an option, we abandon the dying to their suffering. Instead we need to be the sort of community where suicide does not need to be an option, where the dying are not abandoned to the loneliness, pain, and isolation of an intensive care unit but are nurtured, surrounded by loving community, and provided with the means to go through their death with as much care as possible.

	Procedure	Legal Status in United States	Moral Status
Withdrawal of Treatment	Removal of treatment after determination of brain death.	Legally acceptable.	Generally uncontroversial.
	Removal of ventilator from patient in irreversible or terminal condition.	Legally protected right for patient or patient's guardian.	Generally uncontroversial.
	Removal of artificial nutrition and hydration from patient in irreversible or terminal condition.	Legally protected right for patient or patient's guardian.	Condemned by Catholic church, but generally considered acceptable by others.

	Procedure		Legal Status in United States	Moral Status
Euthanasia	Lethal injection used to end the life of a terminal or suffering patient.	Performed at request of patient.	Illegal. (Legally permitted in Netherlands.)	Very controversial, condemned by many churches.
		Performed at request of patient's guardian.	Illegal. (Not legal, but permitted in Netherlands.)	Very controversial, condemned by many churches.
	Physician assisted suicide.	Physician prescribes but may not administer drugs to end patient's life.	Legal in Oregon, illegal elsewhere.	Very controversial, condemned by many churches.

WHAT COUNTS AS DEATH?

Decisions about end-of-life care become particularly acute in the last days and hours of death. Because technology offers the means to keep lungs breathing and hearts pumping well beyond the time when the body could survive on its own, we face the question of when, exactly, death occurs and what counts as death. Doctors use two different standards for determining death. The first, used for most of human history, is that death occurs when the heart and lungs stop irreversibly.

The impetus for a new definition of death came about as a result of organ donation and transplants. In the 1960s, doctors began experimenting with organ transplants. But it wasn't until the 1980s, after the development of the antirejection drug cyclosporine, that doctors began to use these procedures to treat a variety of conditions. When that happened, the demand for organs rose far ahead of the supply.

Using the original definition of death meant that organs used for transplant purposes were often damaged by lack of oxygen during the dying process. Transplant surgeons struggled to obtain organs that were healthy enough to benefit the recipient.

At the same time, patients and families going through end-of-life care were beginning to question the idea that life continues as long as the lungs and heart continue to function. Patients with serious head injuries, for example, could often be kept breathing for days or weeks, even if they had irreversible brain damage and there seemed no hope of restoration of function.

This issue was widely discussed during the Karen Quinlan case. In 1975, Quinlan's family requested that she be taken off a respirator as her brain damage appeared to be irreversible. Her caregivers refused, arguing that taking her off the respirator would be the same thing as killing her. The case went to the New Jersey State Supreme Court, which ruled that the family of a dying patient has the right to decide to let the patient die by removing life support. Quinlan was weaned off the respirator and was transferred to a nursing home until her death in 1986. This case is generally cited as the first case establishing the right of patients and their families to refuse treatment. In the years following the Quinlan case, doctors proposed a new definition of death measured by brain function rather than heart/lung function.

This makes sense. We know that when the brain no longer functions, other bodily functions also cease. We also know that brain function controls much of who we are as persons, including memory, the ability to make decisions, and characteristic responses. From both a social and a physical point of view, then, it makes sense to assume that when the brain no longer functions, the person is no longer living.

In 1981, the American Medical Association and the American Bar Association adopted the Uniform Determination of Death Act. It proposed two sets of criteria, either one of which could be used to determine when someone was actually dead:

▶ The cessation of heart/lung function.
▶ The irreversible cessation of all the functions of the brain, including the brain stem.

Since that time, health care professionals have debated whether the criteria should include the whole brain or just the cortex, and how much electrical activity actually counts as "functioning." But the general principle of whole brain death is widely accepted both in society and by the law as the standard criteria of death.

The debate about how to define death continues, however, in part because of the shortage of organs for donation. In recent years some surgeons have argued for a return to heart/lung criteria in certain cases, because some patients don't meet the criteria for brain death even though they are clearly in the process of dying. In a procedure sometimes called the Pittsburgh protocol—but more accurately called donation after cardiac death—physicians remove a terminal patient from life support, wait until the patient's breathing and heartbeat stop for about five minutes, and declare the patient dead. Then they immediately begin the process of removing organs for donation. Because the timing is so carefully controlled and the patient has undergone some procedures to protect the organs to be donated, the procedure results in usable organs for donation.

This procedure is still controversial. Many caregivers object because it does not seem to focus on the well-being of the patient or the needs of the family. Others worry that it makes the health care system appear too ghoulish, as though doctors are simply waiting for patients to die so they can cannibalize the body. (Many people refuse to sign donor cards because they fear that their bodies will be harvested for organs rather than treated if they end up in an emergency room after an accident.) Those who defend this new protocol argue that it is used only under very carefully specified cases, and only when the family has approved organ donation. (We'll return to the case of organ donation and transplants in chapter 4.)

The media frenzy generated by another famous case has also prompted discussion about brain death criteria. In February 1990, Terri Schiavo suffered a cardiac arrest that resulted in severe brain damage due to lack of oxygen. She was resuscitated at the hospital and eventually moved to a skilled care facility. For several years, Michael, her husband and court-appointed guardian, shared Terri's care with her parents. In 1998 Michael Schiavo petitioned the court for permission to remove his wife's feeding tube. Terri's parents disagreed with this decision very strongly and tried to have Michael removed as her guardian.

One of the issues in the Schiavo case was the question of what it means to be in a persistent vegetative state (see also the sidebar on p. 16). Many people were under the mistaken impression that it is the same thing as brain death. Brain death, however, requires that *all* brain functions have ceased. A person in a persistent vegetative state retains a certain amount of brain function; Terri Schiavo was able to breathe without the help of a ventilator because her brain stem was still functioning. All of the neurologists who examined her agreed that the damage to her brain was irreversible, but the damage did not result in brain death.

The courts decided that Michael Schiavo was an appropriate guardian and that a feeding tube is medical treatment and thus can be removed if the patient or the patient's guardian chooses to remove it.

HOW DO WE DECIDE ABOUT END-OF-LIFE CARE?

In chapter 1 we talked about central aspects of Christian moral reasoning; here we'll think about how these might apply to end-of-life care. We've already noted the place of community in decision-making and the importance of support and prayer in making decisions about the end of life. But we also saw in chapter 1 how our place in the Christian story also has a significant role to play. Death, of course, is one of the most significant events in the story of our life. A life that ends too soon, for example, takes on the aspect of a tragedy. On the other hand, a peaceful death at the end of a long, productive life seems a fitting end to a life well-lived. A death resulting from a heroic sacrifice reminds us of both the tragedy of a life cut short and the courage to make one's death count.

Ultimately, though, we don't determine the stories that provide the structures for our lives. We're called to live as members of the body of Christ, letting the light of God's kingdom shine through our lives. Death usually comes to us in ways we don't choose or control. But how we go through our death is something we may have quite a bit of control over.

As Christians we need to remember that death is part of the life we have been given. Scripture frequently reminds us of our mortality: we are like grass, like flowers that fade. We all die. In contrast, our culture tends to deny the ravages of age. There is a profound tension between a culture that encourages us to hide any signs of aging as if they were shameful and the story of our lives as told by Scripture.

We know that death is not the final word in the story of our lives. Death is an evil, but not the ultimate evil; we rely on God to bear us up and carry us through. And while we mourn death, fight against it, even shake our fists in rage at it, we do not mourn as those who have no hope. Our hope is in the God who created us, who redeems and sustains us.

Death may be the natural end of human life, but it is not a good thing. We know this because the God we worship has overcome death; that is precisely why we hope for eternal life. But we need to hold that hope in tension with an acceptance of our mortality, which is, after all, integral to our humanity.

> "Christianity thus turns out to be not simply about what happens to us after we die, but also about our learning to live together in such a way that our dying—and our caring for others as they die—is the earthly conclusion of a faithfulness we learn and live out along the way."
>
> —Joel Shuman & Brian Volck, M.D., *Reclaiming the Body*

We need to think about how our dying can express our firm commitment to our faith and the life we receive as a gift of God. In this spirit we can fully endorse practices such as hospice that provide resources to help people face their death with courage. We should be more cautious about the frantic grasping at technology to prolong life, no matter what the cost, which suggests that we live by our own efforts rather than by the grace of God. Finally, we should reject practices that welcome or celebrate death such as euthanasia and physician assisted suicide.

Our society isolates the dying in medical facilities, leaving most of their care to strangers. To the extent that the church models a different sort of response—not by taking over the medical role, but by supplementing it with structures of support and love—the church shows what we are called to be as the body of Christ in the world.

Questions for Reflection and Discussion

1. The courts have ruled that a patient has the right to determine his or her own treatment. This means that if someone wants to refuse a treatment that could save her life, she has the legal right to do so. Of course this does not mean it is morally right. Think of some times when Christians should or should not refuse certain treatments, especially life-saving ones. Why or why not?

2. What does your church do to support members and their families when someone is dying? Does the whole church participate in this responsibility, or is it largely the pastor's duty? What may be missing from your church's response?

3. Many Christians believe that euthanasia and physician assisted suicide are always wrong. Should Christians try to make the laws reflect Christian moral beliefs on this subject, or should they accept a separation between secular legal structures and religious beliefs? Why?

For Further Reading

Bregman, Lucy. *Beyond Silence and Denial: Death and Dying Reconsidered.* Louisville: Westminster John Knox Press, 1999.

Bush, Michael D. ed., foreword by Nicholas Wolterstorff. *This Incomplete One: Words Occasioned by the Death of a Young Person.* Grand Rapids, Mich.: Eerdmans, 2006.

Garvey, John. *Death and the Rest of Our Life.* Grand Rapids, Mich.: Eerdmans, 2005.

Spiro, Howard M., Mary G. McCrea Curnen, and Lee Palmer Wandel, eds. *Facing Death: Where Culture, Religion, and Medicine Meet.* New Haven, Conn.: Yale University Press, 1996.

CHAPTER 3

CHRONIC ILLNESS, SUFFERING, AND CHRISTIAN RESPONSES

"Did you hear about the Stewarts' daughter?" Janet asks the women in her Tuesday morning Bible study group. "She's been hospitalized again for depression. Someone needs to tell that girl to get a grip! She's spending far too much time moping around."

"Get a grip!" responds Kathy. "Depression isn't something you get a grip on. Just because it's a mental thing doesn't mean it doesn't need treatment."

"I don't know," adds Mildred. "When my cousin's niece was depressed, they took her to a priest for an exorcism. But then she committed suicide a year later, so I don't think it really worked."

"For heaven's sake!" Janet responds sharply. "Forget the hocus-pocus. What she needs is a bit of old-fashioned willpower. When I get down, I just make sure to keep busy and it always goes away."

Sharon listens quietly. She's been struggling with depression for the last several years. A recent job change makes it likely her medications will no longer be covered by insurance because it's a pre-existing condition. Without the medications she's not sure she can function. One thing is certain—she won't ask this group for prayer support.

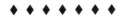

In chapter 2 we focused on end-of-life issues; in this chapter we'll look at chronic illness. These issues are not quite as flashy or as likely to draw media attention as end-of-life cases, but they are far more likely to affect people's daily living. In this chapter we'll consider how the Christian community can respond appropriately and compassionately to those who suffer from chronic illness, whether physical, psychological, or a combination of the two.

Medical care today is divided into two areas: acute care and chronic conditions. Acute care responds to disruptions in a person's normal function—for example, a broken leg, cancer, or a heart attack. When these things happen, patients need immediate diagnosis and treatment. For the most part, we expect the treatment to be a temporary intervention in the patient's life. Either the person gets well again and resumes normal life, or, in the worst-case scenario, the person dies.

Chronic conditions on the other hand—whether diseases like diabetes or bipolar disorder, or chronic pain—are not so much momentary disruptions in people's lives as they are a facet of their lives. These conditions may be present at birth or may come a result of accident or illness. Either way, we too easily identify people by these conditions: "She's disabled," someone might say, or "He's a diabetic." "I'm not disabled," one of my students recently said to me. "I'm a person who has a disability, but that's not my whole identity." When we name people by their condition, there is a strong tendency for us to diminish them to just that condition.

Paradoxically, we need to begin our thinking about chronic conditions by looking at health and the way our understanding of health affects our responses to chronic disease.

HEALTH AND THE LIFE OF THE CHURCH

Our culture treats health as a moral value. It bombards us with messages about things we *should* be doing to protect our health—eating more vegetables, exercising more, managing our stress—and things we *should not* be doing—smoking, gaining too much weight, drinking too much. These messages imply that we are individually directly responsible for our health. The reality is that although we will certainly live better if we are reasonably careful about our lifestyle, most of the conditions that determine our health are a result of genes, environment, and happenstance.

"We claim that people who fail to engage in certain health-promoting activities are generally 'more likely to die,' as though the general risk of dying could be anything less than 100 percent. . . . Such linguistic slips betray a belief that drives the health-seeking behavior of many of us. It is the unspoken, but strong and pervasive, belief that if we just learn enough, do enough, prevent enough, exercise enough, eat the right stuff, purify our air and water and food, none of us will have to die."

—Margaret Mohrmann, *Medicine as Ministry*

The flip side to the idea that we are responsible for our health is that it's our own fault if we aren't healthy. This "blame the unhealthy" mentality is particularly harmful in the context of the Christian community when we suggest that a chronic condition is a result of weak or nonexistent faith, thus adding to the person's pain. It's an attitude Jesus' disciples exhibited centuries ago when they asked of a man who was born blind whether it was his sin or that of his parents that caused the blindness. To their surprise, Jesus responded by saying that the man was born blind "so that the works of God might be displayed in him" (John 9:3).

We can take Jesus' response at face value: the man's blindness offered an opportunity for Jesus to demonstrate who he was—the true Son of God. But there's another lesson in this story: lack of health and chronic illness offer important occasions for us to show God's power and love to the world. Not through dramatic, miraculous healings, but through the way we as the church community respond to those who live with illness.

When we identify health with moral righteousness and individual responsibility, we deny the fact that we will all experience physical illness and dependency at some point. Further, the belief that health is the result of our own moral righteousness allows us to distance ourselves from people with chronic illness. Clearly, such an attitude has no place in the body of Christ.

Our notion of health is always relative to some assumed standard. For example, I can call myself healthy because I've had surgery to remove a ruptured appendix and Lasik surgery to fix profoundly nearsighted eyes and because I take antibiotics to fight regular sinus infections. My health is sustained, in part, by a world that offers the health care I need in an environment that works with my physical capabilities.

The situation of one of my students who uses a wheelchair is different. Because the building where I work was designed for someone with my physical capabilities, I can get around easily. But this same building makes getting around time-consuming, frustrating, and inconvenient for my student. Stairs are everywhere; elevators, on the other hand, are not always placed in convenient spots, and sometimes they don't work at all. The only wheelchair-accessible restroom is on the fourth floor. I am considered healthy because the environment suits my needs; my student is seen as lacking health because the environment doesn't suit his needs. If the environment were designed to accommodate both of us, my student and I would be equally healthy.

"Barriers, both social and physical, prevent people with such deficits from being full members of the community. The irony is that, for many of us as we age, these will be barriers to us too, and our place in 'normal' society will become increasingly hard to maintain."

—Alastair V. Campbell, *Health as Liberation*

But environment is not the only factor in our determination of what we call health. Age plays a role too. We expect a far higher level of activity for a twenty-year-old than for an eighty-year-old. Likewise, cultural expectations change over time. In the 1950s and 60s, for example, it was not uncommon for doctors to prescribe hormones to stunt the growth of tall girls; these days doctors prescribe other hormones designed to increase the height of short children, especially boys. Both cases demonstrate an implicit assumption about what sort of growth pattern and height is "healthy."

Social aspects of health are also affected by cultural assumptions. For example, many theorists point out that the diagnosis of attention deficit hyperactivity disorder (ADHD) is generated in part by the structures of our contemporary society. Societies that do not require children to spend much time sitting quietly don't generally identify hyperactivity as a problem for children.

As we've seen, the concept of "health" is a complex matter that involves physical conditions, social factors, and environmental structures. Chronic health conditions alone need not be incompatible with being healthy. An individual with diabetes or depression can be healthy or unhealthy, depending on whether the condition is controlled or spirals out of control. This too depends partly on environmental and social factors—it is much easier to keep diabetes or depression under control for those who have adequate health care and insurance. Stable family relationships, a decent job, and adequate education all help as well. Ultimately, what counts as health is related to some (often assumed) baseline of our expected capacity to function.

THE COMPLEXITY OF CHRONIC ILLNESS

Like health, chronic conditions are complex. Some chronic conditions primarily affect physical capabilities; others affect a person cognitively, emotionally, and spiritually. Someone who develops paraplegia after an accident, for example, deals primarily with the first sort of chronic condition, while someone who struggles with adult-onset schizophrenia deals with the second.

Chronic conditions that affect primarily physical functioning have no bearing on people's ability to interact with others (though, as we've noted, people who are physically disabled may discover that others sometimes react to them as if they are mentally disabled as well). On the other hand, conditions such as severe depression, bipolar disorder, or schizophrenia are likely to disrupt people's social interactions as well. For example, those with schizophrenia may exhibit antisocial or inappropriate behavior that negatively affects those around them. And when there are no obvious physical signs of illness, it may be harder for people to understand them or feel compassion for them.

Second, we can distinguish between chronic conditions that intrude into a life previously identified as "normal" and those that are present from birth. The onset of Parkinson's disease, for example, affects a person's identity and sense of health differently from the way Down syndrome (which is present from birth) affects a person's identity and sense of health.

Someone who has already established a sense of self is likely to experience the onset of a chronic condition as an attack on her very identity. Coming to terms with this change can result in severe depression, suicidal tendencies, and deep grief, in part because it involves mourning the loss of who the person once was. In contrast, those who are born with a chronic condition are likely to experience it as an integral part of their identity. So when others respond by using negative language like "tragedy" or "defect" to describe the condition, they may feel as though it is an attack on their very right to exist.

In recent years disability rights advocates have responded to prejudice against people with disabilities and lobbied for legislation that would enable them to live healthy, productive lives—including in-home assistance, education, and training for people with special needs. In addition they advocate for a whole range of structures that allow people to move freely and easily through the world, including barrier-free sidewalks and buildings, walk signals with sound indicators in addition to lights, and the like.

DISABILITIES, IDENTITY, AND THE CHURCH COMMUNITY

How can the church community respond to some of these issues? A church that identifies itself as a welcoming community for everyone but has physical barriers that prevent some people from getting in the door is sending decidedly mixed messages. Obviously many older buildings pose accessibility challenges. But the law requires churches to plan for accessibility when they embark on any new construction projects. Churches may unintentionally send similar messages of exclusion in a host of other ways: by emphasizing sports activities in youth groups, by excluding kids with cognitive impairments from Sunday school classes, or by providing wheelchair seating in awkward, out-of-the-way places.

These obvious types of exclusion are relatively easy to address. But a number of other issues are more subtle and may be more difficult for the church to address. Earlier we noted how chronic conditions can affect an individual's identity or sense of self.

"From the very beginning I sensed that my illness represented a fundamental loss of wholeness—a loss of wholeness which related not simply to my physical state but, more importantly, to my personhood. That is, I felt my self diminished along with my body. Our sense of who we are is intimately related to the roles we occupy, professional and personal (wife, lover, secretary, woman, student), and to the goals and aspirations that we hold dear. Chronic, progressive, disabling disease necessarily disrupted (or threatened to disrupt) my every role in ways that, at the outset, seemed to me to reduce my worth as a person. Moreover, the uncertainty of the prognosis transformed my goals and aspirations into foolishness. This sense of diminishment was accompanied by a sense of guilt. I didn't have the energy to do the household chores . . . I needed extra time off from work. . . . In my heart of hearts, I felt in a myriad of ways that I was failing to do as I ought."

—S. Kay Toombs, describing the range of emotional and psychological responses she experiences in her life with multiple sclerosis, from *Chronic Illness: From Experience to Policy*

Many chronic conditions make it difficult to perform basic day-to-day activities. Because our culture glorifies self-sufficiency, most of us find it shameful or embarrassing to ask for help. And in a culture that prizes career success and clear professional goals, many chronic conditions affect people's abilities to make plans for their future. It's easy to see how people with chronic conditions may be distanced from the sorts of activities and experiences that we associate unthinkingly with being an autonomous adult.

In an odd reversal of appropriate roles, people with chronic conditions often find themselves providing emotional support and reassurance to others about their condition. For example, they may be asked to give testimonies about how they've grown spiritually through their conditions. Although honest testimony might sound at times like Job's ("Why did I not perish at birth?" Job 3:11), we often expect to hear uplifting stories. Instead, the church needs to allow those who live with uncertain diagnoses and debilitating conditions to express their grief, anxieties, and frustrations.

Psychological illnesses often go unnoticed, even though they are no less life-changing than physical illness. As the story that begins this chapter illustrates, being able to hide one's condition is a mixed blessing: people may comment on your situation unknowingly. Like Sharon, you may find yourself in the uncomfortable position of having to choose between "coming out" to others or listening to them spread disinformation about your condition. Further, if your condition is not well-controlled by medication, your behavior may seem strange or even morally unacceptable to other people. This raises questions about individual responsibility (Should we blame Mrs. Jones for maxing out all her credit cards during a manic phase?), individual identity (Is it the schizophrenia talking when Sam is being really strange?), and individual autonomy (When is it OK to intervene when Mr. Friedman is drinking again? Or should we just pretend not to notice?).

Chronic psychological conditions can be challenging, exhausting, and frightening. The stigma attached to mental illness is so strong that sufferers will go to extreme lengths to hide their condition, thus making it impossible for others to respond appropriately even if they want to. These challenges are especially acute in the context of the church community because we cannot pretend that we aren't responsible for each other. As the body of Christ, we're commanded to bear one another's burdens and mourn with those who mourn. That means we need to recognize our collective responsibility to respect, love, and support each other, in sickness and in health.

> "The worst thing about mental illness, besides the pain, is this very stigma. The taking pleasure from others' pain. The jokes. Stigma creates a fear on the part of the mentally ill and cycles the fear of those who are healthy against those who are ill."
>
> —Kathryn Greene-McCreight, *Darkness Is My Only Companion*

IT'S ABOUT THE MONEY . . .

People with chronic conditions may be denied insurance coverage or be covered only minimally. In addition, medications are often astonishingly expensive, so people are tempted to do without when money is in short supply. Of course this is costly too: failing to take medications as prescribed can result in the need for stronger or more expensive medications to treat new complications, resulting in an ugly spiral of increasingly difficult medical choices.

But those who live with chronic conditions are not the only ones who bear the enormous financial costs. These costs are shared throughout the health care system. A study carried out by the American Diabetes Association, for example, estimated that in 2007 the cost generated by diabetes care in the United States was $174 billion. Of that, $116 billion was for direct medical expenditures. Add to this the many other conditions people face, and we're faced with truly staggering health care costs. Experts estimate that approximately 80 percent of all health care costs are for chronic conditions.

But our society spends far fewer research dollars on chronic conditions than we might expect. Consider the following example. The National Institutes of Health (NIH) reported that nearly seven million children under the age of eighteen have asthma; the budget for asthma research in 2007 was $294 million. In contrast, the number of people waiting for organ transplants (including kidneys, livers, pancreas or combined pancreas-kidney, heart or combined heart-lung) is just over 100,000 (www.organdonor. gov, 2008); the research budget in 2007 for organ transplants was $357 million. In other words, research money for each child with asthma comes to about $42 per year; for those who need transplants, on the other hand, research dollars add up to about $3,500 for each individual per year.

These numbers are a rough guide to how our health care system distributes research dollars. We spend far more money on acute care and care that affects a relatively small number of people than we spend on chronic conditions that affect large numbers of people. Many economists argue that these priorities are exactly backward: we should spend more money on research into effective treatment for the chronic diseases that affect millions of people and less on drastic and expensive interventions that affect a much smaller number of people. The reality is that research on asthma is neither glamorous nor financially rewarding, while doctors who develop new transplant technologies are venerated by the media.

This economic imbalance takes on a deep poignancy when we know families who face financial ruin as they try to pay for the psychiatric care a loved one needs. Support services for chronic care are effective, but the effects are hard to measure because they keep people out of the health care system. Acute care is much more expensive, but the results are easier to see and publicize. As a result, our health care system provides almost unlimited funds for acute care but inadequate funding for the day-to-day care that makes acute care less necessary.

THE CHURCH AS A COMMUNITY OF CARE

Like the poor, chronic conditions will always be with us. Thus the church needs to be ready to offer Christ's love and support to those who live with various chronic conditions. We've already mentioned the issue of exclusion and access, but because of the specific nature of many chronic conditions, there are many other concrete ways in which the church community can include and provide support for people with chronic conditions.

> "What would a church look like in today's culture if we were to make *shalom* our primary aim? First, it would require us to reorder our values—to put one another and our life together as a community before our personal quests for power, prestige, wealth, and possessions. Second, we would have to drop our façades of independence and self-sufficiency to be vulnerable to one another and support one another in weakness. Third, we would begin to notice the weak and suffering within the church community and to care for them lovingly. Finally, we would reach out in love to the broader community."
>
> —Judith Allen Shelly, *Spiritual Care: A Guide for Caregivers*

We've already mentioned ways that chronic diseases such as multiple sclerosis can affect people's very identity and sense of self. The church community reflects Christ's love to people with chronic conditions when it provides relationships that help people restore their sense of self and when it encourages people to safely express their feelings of fear, frustration, and anger. In addition, the church community can provide regular visits and physical support where appropriate, as well as relief for caregivers.

Of course, different sorts of chronic conditions require different sets of responses. For example, many churches offer Friendship groups, a ministry that is designed to share God's love with people who have cognitive impairments and to enable them to be an active part of God's family (for information and resources on Friendship Ministries, visit www.friendship.org). Other churches provide meeting spaces for a variety of support groups such as Alcoholics Anonymous. Still others provide respite care or financial support for group housing that allows adults with developmental disabilities to live independently. All of these are a wonderful witness to the presence of God's kingdom in the world.

In our culture it is especially easy to feel disconnected with others: we move frequently, we don't know our neighbors, we live far away from family and friends. So the role of the church as a genuine community is more important than ever. And whenever we welcome people into our midst, whenever we provide a haven for the weak and vulnerable, we truly function as the body of Christ in the world.

Questions for Reflection and Discussion

1. How does your church community address the needs of people with chronic conditions? What changes could your church make to be more inclusive in its ministries?

2. What are the factors that shape our assumptions about health? How do these assumptions shape our attitude toward people with chronic illnesses?

3. What role, if any, should the church play in contributing to the conversation about how public dollars are spent for medical research into chronic conditions?

For Further Reading

Cohen, Richard M. *Strong at the Broken Places: Voices of Illness, a Chorus of Hope.* New York: Harper, 2008.

Greene-McCreight, Kathryn. *Darkness Is My Only Companion: A Christian Response to Mental Illness.* Grand Rapids, Mich.: Brazos Press, 2006.

Owens, Virginia Stem. *Caring for Mother: A Daughter's Long Goodbye.* Louisville: Westminster John Knox Press, 2007.

Shelly, Judith Allen. *Spiritual Care: A Guide for Caregivers.* Downers Grove, Ill.: InterVarsity Press, 2000.

Toombs, S. Kay, David Barnard, and Ronald A. Carson, eds. *Chronic Illness: From Experience to Policy.* Bloomington: Indiana University Press, 1995.

Wells, Susan M. *A Delicate Balance: Living Successfully with Chronic Illness.* New York: HarperCollins, 2000.

CHAPTER 4

ORGAN DONATION AND HEROIC MEDICINE

"I really don't know what to do, Doc," says Joseph. "Of course I'm glad I'm a good match for my son, and I think I should donate a kidney to him. He can't live on dialysis much longer—it's impossible for him to work, and his condition is getting worse. But I'm scared too. After all, Jack's not my only kid. Ellen and I have two more—they're still little, and if I were to die, or get kidney failure myself, how would they survive?"

"It's not a simple decision," agrees Dr. Marquez. "That's why we give you the results of the matching tests privately. If people knew you were a match they might put pressure on you, and this is a decision you need to make without pressure. You're a very good match for your son, and he could be on a waiting list for a kidney for a long time, especially since good matches are slightly less common for African Americans. But you're right—the surgery can result in complications, and your loss of a kidney does leave you at a greater risk. I won't pretend this is easy. Could you talk it through with someone you trust, maybe your minister?"

"I'll think about it," Joseph responds. "My Bible study group has been really supportive in the past—maybe their advice and prayers will help. But the more people I tell, the worse I'll feel if I decide not to donate. Talking about it almost seems to force my decision."

"Whatever you decide, I'll support you," says the doctor. "It has to be your decision, and it's got to reflect all the different responsibilities you have. You're right to think of the rest of the family as well as your son. And remember, you can come back to me with any questions you have—I'm happy to share any information you need."

"It's not information I need right now—it's wisdom!" says Joseph, getting up to leave. "And I feel like that's in pretty short supply these days."

◆ ◆ ◆ ◆ ◆ ◆ ◆

Organ transplants are the kinds of medical cases that hit the news. Transplant technologies are tremendously expensive. At the same time, they seem so miraculous and wonderful, and they're so central to our picture of what modern medicine is all about, that it's hard *not* to focus on them! Many of us know of people who have received a heart or a liver transplant that allows them to live for many more years. From the recipient's perspective, organ transplants are a wonderful thing—we even call them "the gift of life" sometimes.

In this chapter we'll look at some of the ethical issues raised by organ donation. We'll see that organ donation represents a particularly potent example of the power of medicine, a power that can generate wonderfully good results but that can also become idolatrous. We'll also look at some principles for developing a Christian response to the use and misuse of technology. In the next chapter we'll move on to questions about access: who gets organs when there aren't enough for everyone who needs them?

ORGAN TRANSPLANTS: A SHORT HISTORY

The idea of transplanting organs has its roots in early attempts at blood transfusions in the 1600s. These attempts sometimes succeeded, but as often as not the patient died. Not until the early years of the twentieth century did scientists discover the various blood types; this, in turn, led to the discovery that some donors and recipients are incompatible. (Rh factors, another compatibility agent, were discovered even later.) These early experiments represent the beginning of the idea that various body parts (not just blood) could perhaps be taken from one person and used for another.

Doctors faced a number of hurdles to organ transplantation, including the ability to identify compatible (or incompatible) antibodies in donor and recipient and keeping donor organs in good enough condition to be transplanted and to connect with the patient's circulatory system. These scientific hurdles pale in significance, though, in comparison to the ethical concerns that arose from the earliest beginnings of organ donation. Although blood or a single paired organ, such as a kidney, can be donated without causing irreparable harm to the donor, most organs are vital to life.

As we mentioned in chapter 2, the ability to provide organ transplants is closely connected with changes in medical care at the end of life. Many donated organs come from people who have been declared brain dead. (In most health care systems, this must be verified by a second examination.)

If the patient and/or patient's family have agreed to donation, doctors remove the organs for transplantation. To prevent any conflict of interest, health care systems require that the physician who pronounces the patient dead cannot be a member of the organ donation team.

Some organs—kidneys, bone marrow, and in some cases, a single lobe of a liver—may come from living donors. For tissues such as bone marrow, the donation offers little risk, but kidney donation includes the risks of major surgery, as well as future health risks if the single kidney should fail.

All transplants involving living donors create a basic conflict of interest: two people who need the same organ. A major ethical concern, then, is to protect donors: they too have a right to medical care focused on their best interests, a right to be protected from pressure, and a right to bodily integrity. Health care systems have developed extensive regulations to prevent the procedure from exploiting the donor. This is one instance in which the difference between the principles of doing good and avoiding harm (beneficence and nonmaleficence) is quite clear. While the former focuses our attention on the recipient of the organ, the latter reminds us that we can never sacrifice the donor for the sake of the recipient.

> Transplant guidelines developed by The United Network for Organ Sharing (UNOS) discourage the use of children as donors, although this sometimes occurs. Ethically, the use of children as donors is especially problematic since they may not understand the long-term risks involved in organ donation.

Thousands of individuals in the United States and Canada are waiting for organs at any given time, and many will die before they receive the organ they need. So when an organ does become available, the recipient feels as though a death sentence has been lifted. The five-year success rate for kidney transplants is between 80 to 90 percent (depending on other health factors and whether the kidney was from a living donor or a cadaver). For heart transplants, the five-year success rate is about 72 percent. Transplant technology, then, offers a very real chance to extend life. For most people who undergo surgery, the chance is worth the risk and the discomfort and expense of antirejection drugs and follow-up care.

MEDICINE AS SAVIOR?

In chapter 1 we noted that medicine is one of the "powers"—it's a societal structure that determines the meaning and direction of significant portions of our lives. Organ transplanting is a category of medicine that clearly fits this definition, especially for those who need a transplant. When organ systems fail and we face death, modern medicine offers a very effective reprieve. No wonder we place our trust in the doctors and nurses who control this powerful force!

> "People will pay anything to defend against the possibility of death, all the more so when the money involved does not come directly out of their own pockets."
>
> —Abigail Rian Evans, *Redeeming Marketplace Medicine*

We tend to remember the positive stories about medicine: a friend close to death whose kidney transplant brought him back to robust health; a baby whose heart transplant allows her to run and play and develop normally. Rarely do we dwell on stories about a failed transplant or a person who dies before an organ becomes available. As a result, we too easily assign medicine the role of savior, the solution to what ails us.

Christians know that any powerful force in human life has the potential for misuse. It is relatively easy to identify individual doctors who misuse their power. It's much harder to recognize and respond to misuse of the power of medicine as a whole. This misuse can happen in two ways. First, medicine itself can misuse the power it wields, resulting in great damage to people and social structures. For example, when medical professionals participated in Nazi Germany's program of euthanizing vulnerable individuals judged "unfit to live," the power of medicine was misused in obvious and hellish ways.

Sometimes, though, it is not medicine that misuses its power so much as people who idolize the power of medicine. Because medicine offers much that is life-giving and good, we are tempted to turn to medicine to solve all our problems. This is especially true with respect to the miraculous interventions offered by modern technology. Describing organ donations, for example, as the "gift of life" slides perilously close to idolatry. Organ transplants can prolong life, and for that we need to thank God. But we shouldn't confuse the extension of life with the source of life, we shouldn't confuse the doctors with God, and we shouldn't expect medicine to offer salvation from our eventual death.

Like any other practice, medicine is a human endeavor. It has the potential to do great good, but it cannot solve all our problems. It is the repository of wonderful knowledge, but no individual's understanding is absolutely perfect. And it is a practice that works with generalities and statistics but applies them to the very particular cases of individuals—which means that it will always fail some time or another.

When medicine fails to live up to its godlike promise, the relationship between doctor and patient becomes one of mutual suspicion and mistrust. The doctor-patient relationship can only be healthy when both participants accept responsibility for what they can do and acknowledge what they cannot do.

"For three decades practicing as a physician, I looked to traditional sources to assist me in my thinking about my patients: textbooks and medical journals; mentors and colleagues. . . . But . . . I realized that I can have another vital partner who helps improve my thinking. . . . That partner is my patient or her family member or friend who seeks to know what is in my mind, how I am thinking. And by opening my mind I can more clearly recognize its reach and its limits, its understanding of my patient's physical problems and emotional needs. There is no better way to care for those who need my caring."

—Jerome Groopman, M.D., *How Doctors Think*

CHRISTIAN DISCERNMENT AND TECHNOLOGY

When evaluating technology, Christians tend to fall into one of two errors. On one hand, Christians are often tempted to reject technology because it involves "playing God" or intervening into matters that should be left alone. On the other hand, we sometimes act as if we can equate technology and scientific advances with salvation. Neither extreme is appropriate.

Our task, then, is to articulate a framework for thinking about medical technologies and their proper place in the life of the Christian community. Let's begin by noting that, like so many other human practices, medical technology is a good gift of God. We know that the "fear of the Lord is the beginning of wisdom" (Prov. 1:7), but we also know that we can turn to the natural world—what John Calvin called the Book of Nature—for wisdom as well. So Christians can legitimately celebrate the work of those who study the wonders of the human body and develop the technologies that can help to repair it.

The second thing to note about technology is that it very often takes on a life of its own. Technological innovations begin by offering exciting new options and end up becoming a requirement. Because we *can* do something, we feel we *must* do it; what started as an option becomes a requirement that involves the need for more money, more resources, and (often) more government oversight. This is called the technological imperative.

Sonograms are a good example. They began as a technology that could be used in cases of high-risk pregnancy to examine the development of the baby. Now they are used routinely in pregnancy—despite the fact that sonograms have not been shown to have any benefit in normally progressing pregnancies. In 1995, the Swiss government decided that state funds would not cover routine ultrasounds because they were unnecessary, but after intense lobbying by pregnant women and their doctors, funds were reinstated. We see here the progression predicted by the technological imperative: sonograms became available, then mandatory; the increase in use resulted in the need for more machines, more money to pay for the procedures, and more involvement by the government.

Our frame of reference as Christians, however, allows us to respond to the technological imperative in another way. We know that technology is not an end in itself; we know we may not turn it into an idol that dictates how our lives should unfold. Our lives, after all, are not our own, but belong in this world and the next to Jesus Christ, our faithful Savior. Further, our response needs to address the way we are called to live together as members of Christ's body. This gives us one important principle for thinking about the use and misuse of technology, a principle emphasized by Joel James Shuman and Keith Meador. Technology is properly used when it protects or restores people to communities of care. Thus, when technology destroys communities, we know that it is not being used properly. As an example, Shuman and Meador point to the way technology often isolates people in intensive care units at the end of life, away from their closest companions.

Technology can also be used to support and protect communities. When we make the benefits of technology available to all members of a community, we signal our recognition that all people, regardless of wealth, class, or disability status, are full members of the community. But when only some have access to technology, we signal that only some people are valued members of the community, while others are second-class citizens. Access to technology thus sends powerful messages of inclusion or exclusion.

In chapter 2 we considered how our pursuit of life-extending technology fits with our professed faith in God as the Lord of life and death. Are we trying to build our own, high-tech tower of Babel, stretching our lives to the very heavens? Or does our pursuit of life-extending technology indicate respect for the fundamental dignity of the image of God in every human? There are no easy answers to these questions. But unless we think through our true goals with respect to these technologies, they may shape us in ways that undermine our Christian faith.

As we noted in chapter 3, our society loves heroic gestures and tends to ignore the quiet, behind-the-scenes work needed to sustain everyday living. Christians, however, bring a different set of values to the world. Our priority should be to serve the weak and vulnerable, to attend to the basic needs of the poor. In so doing we show the world our love for Jesus. So while we can be thankful for what good medicine does, we can also be critical of priorities that run counter to what Scripture reaches.

Finally, we need to realize how the widespread availability of high-tech medicine changes moral relationships. As the story at the beginning makes clear, it has placed additional burdens of responsibility on our shoulders. Before kidney transplants were an option, a loved one's death from kidney failure was a tragic loss—but friends and family had no reason to feel responsible for the death.

Now that transplants are widely available, there is a heavy (if unintentional) burden of responsibility on families and friends. No matter what he decides, a father's decision about donating a kidney to his son may cause grief. If he concludes that his responsibilities to his other children and to his own health are too weighty to run the risks associated with donating a kidney, he may feel responsible for his son's death. But if he decides to donate the kidney, and then suffers health problems of his own, he may feel resentful about having been placed in that situation. We need to share burdens like these with each other as best we can. That means helping each other to think through our responsibilities with prayer and loving support, not judgment or criticism.

Technology continues to change the world we live in. As Christians, we're called to challenge technologies when they conflict with our faith and values, even as we celebrate their potential for good when they restore people to health. In the end, neither superstitious anti-technology nor idolatrous pro-technology responses are adequate—we need thoughtful, prayerful responses that are deeply rooted in the teachings of Scripture and the life of the church.

Questions for Reflection and Discussion

1. In the story that begins this chapter, what advice might you offer to Joseph if he shared the decision he had to make about donating a kidney? Would it make a difference if he were thinking about donating to a friend rather than a son? What about a stranger?

2. What does the development of increasingly complex and expensive technology to lengthen and extend life say about us as a culture? How does our use of (or decision not to use) that technology shape our thinking about our own lives?

3. How can we reconcile our tendency to idolize the incredible medical technologies available to some (but not all) people while at the same time recognizing them as a good gift of God?

For Further Reading

Finn, Robert. *Organ Transplants: Making the Most of Your Gift of Life.* Patient-Centered Guides, 2000.

Kilner, John F., C. Christopher Hook, and Diann B. Uustal, eds. *Cutting-Edge Bioethics: A Christian Exploration of Technologies and Trends.* Grand Rapids, Mich.: Eerdmans, 2002.

Munson, Ronald. *Raising the Dead: Organ Transplants, Ethics and Society.* New York: Oxford University Press, 2004.

Waters, Brent. *From Human to Posthuman: Christian Theology and Technology in a Postmodern World.* Burlington, Vt.: Ashgate, 2006.

CHAPTER 5

SCARCE RESOURCES AND CHRISTIAN COMPASSION

R ob Wisniewski hangs up his phone and sighs. He never dreamed his job as media relations director at Methodist General Health Care System would involve fielding phone calls from TV news outlets asking him to find someone to debate health care issues with anti-immigration groups!

Several months ago, Catholic Immigration Services (CIS) approached Methodist General to arrange care for Lourdes Assuncion, a young girl suffering from kidney failure. Her fifteen-year-old sister is a good match and has offered to donate a kidney; local doctors are willing to perform the surgeries. Methodist General is the only local hospital where kidney transplants are routinely performed, so it's the natural choice. But there's a problem. Lourdes is from Guatemala; she is not a legal resident of this country.

Meanwhile, an anti-immigration group wants Lourdes and her family to be deported. They don't want United States dollars to be spent on providing care for illegal immigrants—not when so many American citizens with no health insurance are going without care. And they want to discuss the matter live, on local television, with a representative from Methodist General.

Rob tries to persuade Dr. Watkins to serve as the hospital's spokeswoman. "I don't know what to think," he says. "How can we let this little girl die when there's a donor kidney available? But on the other hand, how do we justify spending the money when so many citizens can't even afford basic medical care?"

"Seems like the Christian thing to do is to help this kid," replies Dr. Watkins. "Isn't that what the Bible tells us? We're supposed to care for the sick and needy, without regard to their citizenship status."

"Yeah, well, the Good Samaritan only had one person to worry about. We've got an entire county, and pretty limited funds. If we use the money to help this girl, we'll have to turn someone else away. So what does the Bible tell us about that?"

Dr. Watkins grins back. "I have no idea. But I will do the interview for you. Someone needs to speak up for this poor kid."

♦ ♦ ♦ ♦ ♦ ♦ ♦

Medicine, as we noted in the last chapter, can be an enormous force for good—and that very power raises difficult issues. One issue is figuring out who gets access to that healing power, and why, and when. Organ donation offers a particularly difficult case. How do we decide who gets a heart or a liver when there are simply not enough to go around? This is the question of *microallocation*: who gets which specific resources.

But transplant technology also raises more general questions: Is this the best place to focus our efforts when there are so many other types of medical care that cost less and generate greater benefits? These are *macroallocation* questions: how, on a large scale, do we as a society decide to spend the funds we have available for health care? The United States and Canada, for example, have followed different paths in distributing health care. It's worth thinking about how those two different systems look from a Christian perspective.

Let's begin with questions about who is eligible to receive specific resources. We'll use organ transplants as our central example, although the discussion applies to other limited resources as well: beds in intensive care units or nursing homes; respirators, especially if the community faces a serious outbreak of influenza; or access to MRI scanners and other diagnostic tools.

DECIDING WHO GETS WHAT

Donor organs are in very short supply. Over one hundred thousand people are on waiting lists but only around 40,000 organs are donated each year. Why the shortage of donors? For one thing, newer safety regulations (such as motorcycle helmet and seat belt laws) mean fewer people die in accidents now than in the past. (Young, healthy, accident victims offer the best source of organs.) Many people don't sign their donor cards for religious or personal reasons, and even if an accident victim's card is signed, hospitals generally won't harvest organs without the family's consent. Some organs and tissue, of course, can come from living donors (kidneys, bone marrow, sometimes a lobe of a liver), but with the exception of bone marrow, these pose a significant risk to the donor.

When there is simply not enough of any resource to go around, society needs to come up with a system of distribution that allows people to have at least a fair shot at that resource. Putting such a system in place for organ transplants has been extremely difficult. In the early days, transplant decisions were made either by individual doctors or committees formed for that purpose. Both regularly used "social worth" criteria for deciding who deserved the organs: they would favor patients who appeared to be good, worthwhile citizens. People who had professional careers, children, and stable home lives were placed ahead of those who experienced periods of joblessness or who had substance abuse problems or few close family members.

As this system of making decisions came under scrutiny, critics argued that reserving organs for people who meet certain social standards is unfair and unjust. Today health care systems try to use only medical criteria to make decisions about who gets organs. These criteria include general health, blood-type compatibility, and ability to deal with the after-effects of the surgery. (Since transplants require antirejection drugs that can have unpleasant side effects and must be taken regularly, patients need to be capable of keeping to a schedule, or they need family members who will take care of them.) But the line between social and medical criteria is a blurry one. People with stable families are less of a medical risk for transplant follow-up care—so this social issue is medically relevant, as are issues of substance abuse and healthy lifestyle.

Another set of issues revolves around people's ability to pay. In order to be placed on a waiting list, patients need to show that they have the means to pay for the transplant, either by private insurance or some other source of financing. Medicaid covers some transplants in some states but not in others. We've all seen change jars on the counter in convenience stores seeking donations to help pay for a person's transplant fees—an indication of how many folks don't have the financial resources to be eligible for transplants. This raises the same issues as social worth criteria—if it is wrong for people to be excluded from life-saving technology on the basis of social position, isn't it also wrong for them to be excluded on the basis of financial considerations?

Publicity can also factor into the selection process. People who are famous or who have media attention drawn to their case often seem to receive organs ahead of others. In 1995, Mickey Mantle received a donated liver after just two days on the waiting list. This generated intense public debate that was particularly contentious because of Mantle's history of alcohol abuse. In Mantle's case, though, the issue at stake was tissue compatibility. Shortly after his transplant, another liver with a similar tissue match had to be sent elsewhere for lack of a suitable recipient. Even so, the concerns raised in the Mantle case are legitimate—celebrity status should not be a factor in the selection process for receiving organs.

> "Self-destruction is seen by many as its own reward, at least when it comes to booze. Few things can get the blood pressure of the average American up more than finding out that a celebrity alcoholic seems to have snuck to the front of the waiting list for a transplant."
>
> —Arthur L. Caplan, *Am I My Brother's Keeper?*

Still another set of issues arises over the question of whether the selection process should favor those who are the sickest (and so, some argue, the neediest) or those who are healthiest (and thus most likely to be successful candidates and to be able to use the organ for the longest period of time). Arguments can be made on both sides: the sickest are most likely to die without the transplant, but to deny healthier candidates an organ and give it to someone so sick that they don't survive the surgery seems morally problematic.

Today organ allocation is governed by a set of guidelines created by the United Network for Organ Sharing (UNOS). This organization was created to make organ allocation fairer and more transparent and to coordinate organ transportation in a reasonable manner. Because time and distance make a difference, the closer one is, geographically, to a donated organ, the better the chance of a successful transplantation. UNOS provides information about organ transplant policies, sponsors public debate, and ensures accountability for the whole process.

DIFFICULT DECISIONS ABOUT RESOURCES

The policymakers of UNOS are responsible for establishing a fair set of guidelines to govern access to organs. But an important, broader question remains. Should we try to provide organ transplants to all who could benefit from them? Is this really the best policy for United States medicine?

Commentators sometimes note that medicine is a victim of its own success. Most businesses go bankrupt because they aren't very good at what they do; medicine risks going bankrupt because it is very, very good at what it does. We see this dynamic at work in the field of organ transplants. Before transplants were widely available, people with organ failure would die. The medical costs of end-of-life care were fairly limited. Now a person with end stage renal disease can be kept alive indefinitely on dialysis or can receive a kidney transplant (the success rates for kidney transplants are very high). The cost of dialysis is, on average, $65,000 per year. Kidney transplant surgery costs about $102,000, and the cost of antirejection drugs and follow-up care ranges from $6,000 to $10,000, depending on other complications such as diabetes.

When the treatment was less effective, people with kidney disease generated fairly few expenses. Now that far better treatments are available, the expenses associated with renal disease have skyrocketed. And this is true of almost every area of health care. The better we get at offering high-technology treatments for health problems, the more people will use them, and the less we can all afford health insurance.

At the same time that these high-tech interventions for relatively few people are generating skyrocketing health care expenses in the United States, millions of people lack basic care (including prenatal care and regular checkups). For society as a whole, basic care is far more effective in terms of dollars spent.

These broader issues will not go away any time soon. As Christians we should have a voice in the national conversation about health care. Our concern for justice prompts us to think through what sorts of health care our society should provide for all its members. Certainly some level of basic care should be available for everyone. At the same time, recognizing that resources are finite, and that we also need to provide services such as police protection, education, and environmental oversight for the public good, we also need to be realistic about the limits of the care we can provide.

> "Scarcity cannot be denied; we simply do not have the resources to do all we can do, or all we want to do, for all patients. Scarcity requires a limit to what a community provides, but a just compassion requires that in allocating scarce resources we *first* secure access to an adequate level of care for *all*."
>
> —Allen Verhey, *Reading the Bible in the Strange World of Medicine*

The idea that all members of society deserve some basic level of health care raises two difficult questions. First, what is that basic level of health care? Whatever level we decide upon, we are certain to face difficult issues when individuals want and need more care but don't have the money to pay for it. Using citizen focus groups and extensive statewide discussions, the state of Oregon tried to define basic care for its citizens and settled on a list of medical treatments that could be offered to all citizens. They also had to decide which treatments would not be covered—and liver transplants were among them. Within a year, a young boy whose family had a very low income needed a liver transplant. Without it he was sure to die. At first the state refused to pay, but the public was outraged and the operation was covered.

This worked out well for the boy who needed a liver. But it did not work so well for the many Oregonians who then lost insurance coverage because the state could no longer afford to provide care for all. The fact is that individual life-or-death cases often capture enough media attention to determine policy without any careful discussion about what that change in policy means for thousands of other people.

The second difficult question raised by the idea of basic care concerns the definition of membership in the community. We in the United States can be justly proud of our heritage as a nation of immigrants. But many citizens object to providing medical care for immigrants, regardless of their legal status, and several states have passed legislation prohibiting Medicaid care for immigrants. This is hard to justify from a Christian perspective. Deuteronomy 24 reminds us that the poor and needy, whether citizens or aliens, are to be treated justly.

A just legal system should take account of the differences between legal immigrants, illegal immigrants, and citizens. But whatever policies we as a nation put in place to respond to the medical needs of legal or illegal immigrants, the Christian community must speak out against unjust or vicious responses. Immigrants are fellow imagebearers of God, and we can never justify treating them as anything less.

It is interesting to compare the results of health care systems that provide care for all their citizens (Canada and Great Britain, for example), and those that use mixed systems of government funding, private insurance, and the free market to distribute health care, such as the United States. Most free market proponents argue that any system of universal health care would be far more expensive than a free market system. But analysis of health care in these countries does not bear this out: although both Canada and Great Britain and spend quite a bit less, per capita, than the United States, their health care (measured in terms of infant mortality, longevity, and the like) is slightly better. Both the Canadian and British systems limit access to a variety of procedures, either in the form of lengthier waits for some procedures or more stringent limitations on who qualifies for certain transplant procedures. Americans have not traditionally been willing to accept such limits to access.

As we've seen, the fair allocation of health care raises difficult questions from a Christian standpoint. On the one hand, we should be critical of a sense of entitlement and the demand for all the latest technology. On the other, we are to be concerned with providing care for everyone. As a society, our answers to these questions say much about which people we value—and which we do not.

CONCLUSION

Contemporary high-tech medicine is a wonderful gift for which we can thank God. At the same time, it raises unexpected and very difficult questions about what sorts of treatment we can fund, for whom, and under what circumstances. These are difficult questions because the answers may not be the ones we want to hear. Remembering that it is not medicine that provides our lives with meaning and salvation allows us to keep these issues in perspective as we try to address them as a community. One thing is sure: there are no easy answers when it comes to deciding whether to fund basic care for chronic conditions or high-tech care for extreme conditions. We don't have enough resources to provide both, and either answer leaves someone without needed care.

But we do know that Christians are called to speak up for the most vulnerable in our society and to make sure that their needs are met. As a society, we may freely debate and reason together about these matters. As hard as that conversation may be, it is one we need to engage in humbly, prayerfully, lovingly, and honestly.

Questions for Reflection and Discussion

1. If you were asked whether Christians should be in favor of providing health care for illegal immigrants, what would you say? How do we balance our duty toward our fellow citizens with the Christian call to love our neighbors as ourselves?

2. One of the most difficult issues in organ allocation is whether to give preference to the sickest patients (who are less likely to survive surgery) or to healthier patients (who are more likely to survive surgery and to live longer). What basic Christian principles can help us, as a society, address this conflict?

3. Countries such as Canada and Great Britain have made different choices about providing basic health care to all their citizens than the United States has. Why is it important for Christians to participate in the debate about limited resources? What are some of the implications of our choices for society as a whole?

For Further Reading

Daniels, Norman and James Sabin. *Setting Limits Fairly: Can We Learn to Share Medical Resources?* Oxford: Oxford University Press, 2002.

Herzlinger, Regina. *Who Killed Health Care? America's $2 Trillion Medical Problem—and the Consumer-Driven Cure.* New York: McGraw-Hill, 2007.

Kilner, John F., Robert D. Orr, and Judith Allen Shelly, eds. *The Changing Face of Health Care: A Christian Appraisal of Managed Care, Resource Allocation, and the Patient-Caregiver Relationships.* Grand Rapids, Mich.: Eerdmans, 1998.

Relman, Arnold. *A Second Opinion: Rescuing America's Health Care.* New York: PublicAffairs, 2007.

CHAPTER 6

ABORTION

L uke Striker, a junior in college, has been missing a lot of classes lately. Now he's sitting in Professor Johnson's office to explain what's going on.

"I'm sorry about the missed classes," he says, taking a deep breath. "This is hard for me to talk about. You see, my girlfriend is pregnant. I've been driving back to see her and talk about what we're going to do, and then we had to tell our parents. I'm dropping out of college, and then we're getting married in a month or two. It's been really hard."

"Wow—that's a tough situation," Professor Johnson replies. "It sounds as though you're dealing with it with a lot of maturity, though. I'm really sorry to hear you're dropping out of school. You've been doing well in class up to now—and a college education is important."

"Yeah, but I've got to support a wife and kid. I need a full-time job. Maybe I can pick up a few courses—night school or something—at the community college. And my dad got me a job offer."

"I hope your families are proud of you for making hard decisions like this," says his professor. "Lots of kids choose abortion as an easier way out."

Luke's eyes fill with tears. "You know—that's one of the hardest things about this whole deal. We could have, but we didn't. Sometimes I wish we had. Because all we're hearing is what a disappointment we are to our families. Life looks pretty miserable right now."

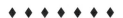

In this chapter we move to the intensely personal issue of abortion and the complex public policy questions it raises. We will describe the different positions Christians have taken on this issue and their reasons for choosing those positions. We'll also examine the effect of abortion on women's lives and wonder whether there are places where those who disagree on abortion may find common ground for policies and specific actions. Finally, the chapter looks at how the church can address this issue as the body of Christ.

CHRISTIAN PERSPECTIVES ON ABORTION

All those who represent official church positions agree that abortion is a tragedy. Nonetheless, various denominations and theologians approach the issue in different ways. On one end of the spectrum, the Roman Catholic Church prohibits its health care systems from providing any "material cooperation" with procedures that involve abortion or sterilization, both of which are treated in the same category. The Catholic Church prohibits abortion even when necessary to save the mother's life. Many other churches hold the view articulated by the Christian Reformed Church that abortion is always wrong and may be considered only when the mother's life is threatened (see sidebar).

> "Because the CRC believes that all human beings are imagebearers of God, it affirms the unique value of all human life. Mindful of the sixth commandment—"You shall not murder" (Ex. 20:13)—the church condemns the wanton or arbitrary destruction of any human being at any stage of its development from the point of conception to the point of death. The church affirms that an induced abortion is an allowable option only when the life of the mother-to-be is genuinely threatened by the continuation of the pregnancy."
>
> —CRCNA Position Statement on Abortion. To read the full statement, visit http://www.crcna.org/pages/positions_abortion.cfm.

A slightly more permissive perspective is found in the work of theologian and bioethicist Gilbert Meilaender. He argues that while a woman may choose to continue a pregnancy that either threatens her life or is the result of incest or rape, Christian theological considerations do not make an abortion under such conditions unacceptable.

A bit further along this spectrum is the position of theologian and bioethicist Allen Verhey. Verhey argues that the range of Christian views on abortion, like the range of Christian views on killing in war time, is fairly broad. For pacifist Christians who believe all killings are incompatible with the law of love, an absolute ban on abortions is consistent. But for Christians who recognize the legitimate use of violence under certain conditions such as war or self-defense, for example, consistency suggests that the violence of abortions can be justified by similarly weighty considerations.

The Presbyterian Church (USA) holds the view that, while abortion is always to be mourned, it may, on occasion, be the lesser of two evils (see sidebar). Voices even further along this spectrum include theologians Daniel Maguire and Beverly Wildung Harrison, who argue that women's legal access to abortion is compatible with Christian principles.

"The considered decision of a woman to terminate a pregnancy can be a morally acceptable, though certainly not the only or required, decision. Possible justifying circumstances would include medical indications of severe physical or mental deformity, conception as a result of rape or incest, or conditions under which the physical or mental health of either woman or child would be gravely threatened."

—PC(USA) Position Statement on Abortion. To read the full statement, visit http://www.pcusa.org/101/101-abortion.htm

The range of views on this subject is wide (see table on next page); the passions felt by various advocates are strong; the potential for divisive and adversarial interactions enormous.

Lisa Sowle Cahill notes that people talking about abortion tend to use two different types of "voices." Public debates between the pro-choice and the pro-life advocates adopt a single voice, or type of language— Cahill calls it "prophetic discourse." This voice emphasizes the use of slogans and simplistic images. It serves primarily to reinforce bonds within the group of like-minded people, and it widens divisions between those who disagree.

"In national debate activists usually come from partisan groups that have a fervent ideological commitment or a large economic stake in a polar outcome of the issue. Therefore, the primary speakers on any issue are generally unwilling to listen to the other side or to reach caring compromises, and they are tempted to turn to coercion to gain their ends."

—Celeste Michelle Condit, *Decoding Abortion Rhetoric*

RANGE OF VIEWS ON ABORTION

Reason for Abortion	Legal Status in U.S.	Moral Status
Pregnancy puts woman's life at risk	Legally permitted at all stages of pregnancy.	Accepted as legitimate by most Christians, condemned by Catholic Church.
Pregnancy puts woman's health at risk	Legally permitted at all stages of pregnancy.	Accepted as legitimate by some Christians, rejected by others.
Pregnancy result of rape/incest	Not specifically addressed in most abortion rulings.	Accepted as legitimate by some Christians, rejected by others.
Severe fetal abnormalities (anencephaly, Tay-Sachs disease)	Legally permitted at all stages of pregnancy.	Accepted as legitimate by some Christians, rejected by others.
Moderate fetal abnormalities (Down syndrome, hemophilia)	Legally permitted at early stages of pregnancy, legality varies from state to state in later stages.	Generally considered unacceptable by most Christians.
Social circumstances (abusive relationship, economic hardship)	Legally permitted at early stages of pregnancy, legality varies from state to state in later stages.	Controversial—condemned by many Christians, defended by some.

The other kind of voice we can use to speak about the issue encourages thoughtful dialogue and consensus building. This voice is characterized by listening before pronouncing. It examines the ways women experience abortion, the reasons they choose abortion, and the ways that social policies—including abortion laws, welfare policies, and legal protection against violence and abuse—affect women's experiences of pregnancy and childbearing. This voice recognizes that women have abortions in countries with liberal abortion laws as well as those that prohibit abortions; and they do so even under unsafe conditions that can lead to death. This kind of desperation suggests that abortion is much more than a question about legality. More broadly, it is a question about women's place in society, their relationship with children, and their relationship with the men who are also responsible for their pregnancies.

ABORTION: THE PERSONAL DIMENSION

Most of us know someone who has had an abortion. But we may not know who that person is. Especially in Christian circles, the stigma of abortion runs deep, and women who have had or have considered having an abortion are unlikely to speak of it publicly. Even though many women are reluctant to speak about their personal experiences, statistics and studies of women who have abortions offer a window into the factors that lead women to consider abortions.

The authors of an anthology titled *Bitter Fruit* have collected stories from women with unwanted pregnancies. Some had abortions, some gave their babies up for adoption, and others kept their babies. These stories sound nothing like the political rhetoric surrounding the topic of abortion; there is very little of the language of "rights." Rather these are the stories of very scared young women facing almost insurmountable complexities. Many of them have emotionally or physically abusive sexual partners. Many have been exposed to violence and neglect in their families. The women who have abortions often grieve them, as do the women who gave their babies up for adoption. Women in both categories talk about how the experience alienated them from their religious communities.

Unfortunately, public discussion about abortion often takes place in isolation from the other issues that are connected with women's decisions about abortion and adoption: issues such as sexuality, welfare, violence against women, and health care funding. During debates in the 1990s about welfare reform, for example, the question of whether families with more children should receive larger monthly assistance payments became a central item of contention. Some conservatives argued that larger payments encouraged single mothers to have more children in order to get larger monthly checks. Their opponents argued that failing to provide extra help when a mother has extra mouths to feed encourages women to abort rather than carry their children to term. When money is scarce, an extra mouth to feed may mean that the family loses its housing. Studies show that there is, in fact, a correlation between the family cap and increased abortion rates. Thus phrases like "protection of life" ring hollow when paired with policies that punish women who give birth.

> "In the construction of the public debate, women's actual lives and experiences have figured very little. When women themselves talk about their own abortion decisions, the unambiguous, polarized rhetoric of the public debate fades and a different experience emerges. Women's statements are highly conflicted and deeply ambivalent."
>
> —Christine Pohl, *Bioethics and the Future of Medicine*

A significant number of abortions are sought by women in emotionally and physically abusive relationships, or who are the victims of rape or incest. Some of these abortions are a result of pressure from the abusive partner (abusive men may become more aggressive when a woman is pregnant). Others may occur because a woman fears that having a child will make it much harder to escape the abusive relationship. One study of married women who obtained abortions found that one in four reported spousal rape or battering. A recent article in the Canadian Medical Association Journal noted that abuse rates are not only high among pregnant women (and directly correlated with health risks for babies); they also correlate with women who cite relationship problems when they request pregnancy termination. Treating the issue of abortion in isolation from these facts about women's lives is irresponsible.

MORAL VALUES: A REVIEW OF THE DEBATE

Debates about the moral status of abortion tend to emphasize either the nature of the fetus or the woman's right to make reproductive choices. Let's begin with a quick review of the last thirty years of the debate.

Those who argue that abortion is morally wrong usually begin by saying that the fetus is fully human from the moment of conception (for example, see the sidebar on p. 66, an excerpt of the position of the Christian Reformed Church). When a sperm and egg join, the resulting embryo (a single cell) has a new genetic code and the potential to go through all the developmental processes that mark the beginnings of each human life. This position holds that anything we might do to prevent that embryo from going through those developmental processes is just as wrong as ending the life of any other human. Morally they are the same.

Many thinkers point out some theoretical and practical weaknesses of this argument. Referring to the "moment" of conception, for example, is problematic since the merging of the sperm and egg is a process that takes several hours to complete. So if we accept that conception marks the beginning of human life, there is a period of time when we aren't sure whether or not the entity we are concerned with counts as a human life. But this criticism is relatively minor.

More serious criticisms point to the various processes of development that an embryo must go through and argue that it would be more accurate to speak of it as a potential person than an actual person. The two processes that have tended to get the most attention in the debate are twinning and implantation. We'll start with implantation.

Implantation

Under normal conditions of conception, the egg and sperm meet, and fertilization takes place in the woman's fallopian tube. (Women have two fallopian tubes, each one of which provides a conduit from one ovary to the uterus.) The fertilized egg then travels down the fallopian tube for a few days to the uterus where, in most cases, it implants into the uterine wall. Implantation involves the development of an intricate interrelationship between the embryo and the woman's body. These include hormonal interchanges and the eventual growth of connections between the woman's circulatory system and that of the developing fetus—connections that are made in the placenta. The process takes some time, and there are a number of points when it may fail. When fertilized eggs do not implant, they simply fail to develop.

Because of this uncertainty and potential for failure, some have argued that a fertilized egg by itself does not have the potential to become a human being. Since an embryo needs to be implanted before it has the full potential to develop into a human being, they believe implantation, not fertilization, should be the marker that identifies full human life.

The question of whether implantation should be considered significant is not just academic. Infertility clinics regularly produce embryos that are not implanted. Usually these are either discarded or frozen for later use; many of the latter are never implanted. If the failure to bring an embryo to fruition is the same as murder, one could argue that infertility clinics destroy human life as much as abortion clinics. However, many people who consider themselves pro-life use the services of infertility clinics. One way of resolving this apparent contradiction is to consider implantation more significant than fertilization, defining the beginning of human life as the joining of a fertilized egg with the uterine support system.

Twinning

The issue of twinning also arises in debates over the status of embryos. For some time after implantation, the developing zygote has the potential to split and become two developing beings. (This is the origin of identical, but not fraternal, twins. Fraternal twins occur when two eggs are each fertilized and implant at the same time.) The phenomenon of twinning poses a real puzzle about whether the embryo can be considered a unique human being—if there are two unique human beings who can trace their existence back to that single cell, one can hardly say that the cell is one unique human being. (Logic seems to preclude such a statement.) Since we don't know which embryos will develop into one person and which into two, some have argued that any embryo is, at best, a potential source for one (or two) human beings rather than a unique human being.

Potentiality versus Actuality

Finally, the issue of the status of the fetus is complicated by the notion of potentiality versus actuality. Some have argued that while a fetus does not yet have all the characteristics of a fully formed human being (fetuses cannot think, for example, nor can they communicate or make plans about their lives), it is potentially a human being and therefore must be treated with the respect due a potential human. In this view, terminating a pregnancy is not the same as killing a fully developed human being. It is, nonetheless, a very grave wrong because we are to protect also the potential for a human life.

You may have noticed that so far this discussion has focused almost exclusively on the status of the fetus or embryo. As we've already pointed out, arguments against abortion tend to be carried out without much focus on the woman involved.

Those who argue in favor of accepting abortion under some circumstances, on the other hand, tend to focus on the pregnant woman. Some of these deny the personhood of the fetus altogether, choosing instead to emphasize the individual autonomy—the right to make choices about our own life—that our society values so highly. If we accept that the embryo or fetus is not a person, then a decision to end a pregnancy does not involve a conflict between one person's right to life and another's right to control her body.

Others argue that even if we accept that the fetus is a person with a right to life, it may still be the case that a woman has the right to terminate certain types of pregnancies, for example, a pregnancy she has not consented to. This argument makes a distinction between a person's right to life, and his or her right to use someone else's resources to preserve that life. For example, while a woman has a right to life, she doesn't have the right to demand that someone donate a kidney if she is in acute renal failure. Similarly, if a woman chooses not to let a developing fetus use the resources of her body, she has the right to terminate the pregnancy.

Note that these arguments focus on the woman and tend to set aside the developing embryo or fetus. Abortion is a complex and difficult moral issue precisely because it is not just about individuals or individual rights. It's about two lives that are interrelated. Women who become pregnant generally call their developing fetus a baby. But they also face agonizing decisions about carrying out the responsibility of mothering a child in a world that doesn't provide much support for that process; perhaps even as part of a religious community that characterizes single mothers as lazy and shiftless, uncaring and irresponsible. Faced with social disapproval and perhaps with a lack of support or access to decent child care, it is not surprising that many women choose abortion as the least of a host of evils, even though they may come to regret their decision profoundly and struggle with it all their lives. This is true even for women who choose abortion as a result of rape or incest.

As Christine Pohl points out in her perceptive discussion of the complexities of abortion decisions in women's lives, framing abortions as a matter of private choice makes it easy to keep the complexities of the decision out of sight and away from the rest of the community. Abortion, she says, "provides a significant escape from responsibility—not just for the woman, but also for the male participant, larger family, church, and economic and political spheres. In a diabolical way, abortion suggests itself to many as the easiest way out of unexpected pregnancies for all involved." Moral debate too often oversimplifies the complexity of women's decisions about abortion and overlooks the morally tragic aspects of these decisions in women's lives.

THE CHURCH AS WITNESSING COMMUNITY
While abortion is likely to remain an issue about which people disagree deeply, the Christian community need not be a source of hate-filled rhetoric or divisiveness. How can Christians bring a gospel of grace in the context of the abortion debate, which is characterized more by name-calling and verbal attacks than by love, gentleness, or longsuffering? The church's witness needs to reflect the attitude Jesus himself adopted in his ministry—an attitude of compassion and responsiveness.

In her book *Theological Bioethics*, Lisa Cahill proposes a balance on which Christians across the spectrum of views on abortion should agree. "Religious leadership against abortion will only have oppressive consequences to . . . women," she argues, "unless it comes in the form of strong, consistent advocacy for women's overall well-being, formulated in dialogue with women themselves." As Christine Pohl puts it, "being pro-life will involve much more than being anti-abortion. Being pro-life requires thoughtful attention to the context of abortion decisions—to the structural arrangements and relationships that leave abortion looking like the easiest and most responsible choice."

> "When I speak to church-sponsored meetings and seminaries about abortion, ministers and seminarians often try to convince me that they already are supporting women with unwanted pregnancies in their churches. When I ask what that support looks like, they tell me they bring such women bags of groceries or send a small check. These well-meaning Christians often cannot understand why more women in their parishes don't choose adoption rather than abortion."
>
> —Kathy Rudy, *Beyond Pro-Life and Pro-Choice*

In addition to participating in the abortion debate, the church is called to show Christian compassion and to offer support to those experiencing unwanted pregnancies as well as to those who have undergone abortions. This compassionate response must include ministry that extends the gospel of forgiveness and grace to women who have had abortions so they can deal with their deep wounds and guilt.

When our focus in the Christian community is less on attacking the arguments of those we disagree with and more on how we can work together to provide real options and social support for women who face unwanted pregnancies, we show the world what it means to be the body of Christ. Such a response includes two components. The first concerns relations within the church and our responsibility to treat fellow Christians charitably and honestly. Demonizing anyone who disagrees with us on the topic of abortion will not lead to a cohesive community, even though it may make us feel righteous and self-satisfied. We need to listen to and engage others with respect, even when there is disagreement, and live with them as brothers and sisters even as we disagree.

The second and more important component of such a response concerns providing an alternative to our culture's perspective on having children. We live in a culture that makes having children a heavy burden on many women. Although most women (and men) love their children and make great sacrifices for them, our culture increasingly treats children as expensive indulgences. Single mothers are not respected for the sacrifices they make and the overwhelming burdens they bear—instead they are described as one of the most significant social problems of our day. We have privatized the raising of children to such an extent that we assume that parents don't deserve help when they struggle—ignoring the fact that raising children is the responsibility of the whole community, as well as the fact that the children who are neglected today will be the adult citizens on whom our community depends tomorrow.

As Christians we need to reject this privatized view of children and offer an alternative vision of communal responsibility for the support and loving guidance of the children among us. When the church community provides day care services so mothers can work and support their families, when the church supports the work of safe houses that protect women from violence and abuse, when churches come together to provide cars or other transportation for women struggling to stay afloat financially, its concern for the lives of unborn children carries weight in the debate about abortion. And when the church community insists that society has a responsibility to care for children growing up in poverty, and that punitive measures toward women who have babies are unacceptable, then its claims to care for all human life will not sound like empty rhetorical gestures.

Scripture affirms that the way we treat those who are most vulnerable—including, certainly, those who are unborn—is a measure of justice (see Isaiah 1:15-17; James 1:27). As the church affirms the unique value of all human life, and as it works to protect the most vulnerable members of society, we honor God's gift of life. But our witness to the world about the sanctity of human life is credible only when it is matched with actions that show our compassion to women who have had abortions or who face the daunting task of raising children on their own.

Together,
male and female,
single and married,
young and old—
every hue and variety of humanity—
we are called to represent God,
for the Lord God made us all.
Life is God's gift to us,
and we are called to foster
the well-being of all the living,
protecting from harm
the unborn and the weak,
the poor and the vulnerable.

—Paragraph 11, *Our World Belongs to God: A Contemporary Testimony*, www.crcna.org/pages/our_world_main.cfm.

As members of the church, we need to welcome those in our midst. We need to bear each other's burdens so that pregnancy need not be an insurmountable barrier to a decent human life, so that single-parent families or families with children who have severe disabilities do not face impoverishment or ostracism, and so that the world sees an alternative to treating children as private luxuries. In the context of a community focused on living as God's people in the world, it is possible for Christians to address the deeply difficult issue of abortion with love for each other and with reverence toward human life.

Questions for Reflection and Discussion

1. This chapter lists several ways the church can show its support for women facing unwanted pregnancies. What activities does your church engage in that make it a supportive community for women facing unwanted pregnancies? Can you think of other ways to strengthen the church's witness to the gift of human life?

2. How are some of the ways we talk about abortion helpful or harmful to the discussion?

3. Imagine that a member of your congregation has come to you to ask for prayer. She is considering having an abortion because her baby has severe anomalies and will not survive once it is born. What considerations should she take into account in this case? Could she bring this difficult decision to others in the church for prayer and community support?

4. How can the church extend the gospel of God's grace and forgiveness to those who have had abortions? Why is this an important part of the church's participation in the debate about abortion?

For Further Reading

Hui, Edwin C. *At the Beginning of Life: Dilemmas in Theological Bioethics.* Downers Grove, Ill.: InterVarsity, 2002.

Kilner, John F., Nigel M. de S. Cameron, and David L. Schiedermayer, eds. *Bioethics and the Future of Medicine: A Christian Appraisal.* Grand Rapids, Mich.: Eerdmans, 1995.

Rudy, Kathy. *Beyond Pro-Life and Pro-Choice: Moral Diversity in the Abortion Debate.* Boston: Beacon Press, 1997.

CHAPTER 7

ASSISTED REPRODUCTION
AND EMBRYO SELECTION

Gina and Simon Brown are nervously waiting for a report in the office of Dr. Pascale at the Westside Clinic for Assisted Reproduction.

"I've got good news and bad news for you," Dr. Pascale announces. "The eggs we harvested and fertilized last month have been tested. We have two embryos, but one shows a genetic abnormality—Down syndrome. That leaves us with just one viable embryo. We could freeze that one, go through another round of egg harvesting, and try for a few more. Your chances of a successful pregnancy are higher with more than one embryo to implant."

"Didn't you tell us four eggs were harvested, though?" Gina asks. "That procedure wasn't really pleasant, with all the hormones and cramping. If I have to go through that again, maybe get another viable embryo, and then wait for my regular cycles to resume—we're talking a lot of time and money. We've already been trying for two years, and we thought this would be the last thing we'd try."

"Well, we can try for implantation with just the one embryo," Dr. Pascale responds, shaking her head. "But chances are just lower with only one. We really prefer to implant at least two. It's unfortunate that only two eggs were fertilized, and that the one embryo is abnormal. But you're so close at this point—it would be a shame to stop now."

As they leave the office and head toward their car, Gina asks Simon, "What should we do? Try again? Try to implant just the one embryo? Or what?"

"I don't know," Simon responds. "We're already past what we planned to spend, and it feels like this is eating up our life. But when I think about stopping and not having a baby . . . well, that just hurts. I don't know what to think. I can't figure out whether it's incredibly selfish of us to spend all this money, or whether trying so hard to have a child shows how unselfish we are."

◆ ◆ ◆ ◆ ◆ ◆ ◆

Many Christians use various techniques of assisted reproduction, some of which are relatively unproblematic. Others raise serious ethical concerns. In this chapter we'll consider infertility treatments that seem problematic and discuss the ethical ramifications of embryo selection, including how that intersects with the abortion issue. Finally, we'll raise questions about issues connected with assisted reproductive technologies.

In chapter 5 we noted that technology is never completely neutral. New technology changes the choices we have to make, it changes our perception of normalcy and abnormality, and it affects our interpersonal relationships. Few areas demonstrate this truth more obviously than assisted reproduction. In the past, couples who were unable to have children had to deal with their emotional reactions to infertility but they did not face emotionally exhausting decisions about how much time and money and energy to spend on pursuing their goal of a successful pregnancy. Nor did they have to face questions from well-meaning relatives about why they did not pursue other medical options. Further, parents with a family history of genetic disorders face questions today that they never would have had to deal with fifty years ago: Is it irresponsible to have a child without undergoing testing? Should the fetus be tested? The presence of new technologies changes our lives and it changes our moral responsibilities.

We'll begin with a brief look at what sorts of technologies are now available, and what sorts of values these new technologies embody. Some of these values—such as compassion for people who want children but are infertile—are compatible with Christian principles. Other values are not—such as the belief that any technology, no matter what risks it poses to a mother or child, is acceptable as long as it achieves the desired result.

ASSISTED REPRODUCTIVE TECHNOLOGIES (ART)

People who want assistance in reproduction can choose from a range of options. In vitro fertilization (IVF), the so-called "test-tube baby" technique many of us think of with respect to assisted reproduction, was first used successfully in the late 1970s. It resulted in the birth of Louise Brown.

> In vitro fertilization involves fertilization outside the body (in a Petri dish rather than a test tube) after which the embryo is replaced in the woman's uterus (or, in some techniques, the fallopian tube) in the hope that the embryo will implant and the woman will go through a normal pregnancy and delivery.

Because IVF separates the various aspects of normal procreation into distinct steps, this technology has led to a broad variety of assisted reproductive techniques at various points in the process. The sperm and egg brought together for fertilization, for example, can be those of the couple involved, or one or the other can be from someone else. (Usually the other person is called a "donor." This term is inaccurate, since these transactions usually involve payment.) Some clinics offer embryos for purchase as well. Because fertilization occurs outside the body, it is also possible for the gestational mother (the one who carries the baby to term) to be different from the egg donor and/or the mother who will raise the child. We'll return to surrogacy issues later.

Because infertility can result from a number of different factors, infertility clinics offer a variety of techniques in addition to IVF. In cases where the man's sperm count is low or the sperm lack the mobility to fertilize the egg in the usual way, clinics may use a technique called intracytoplasmic sperm injection (ICSI) to inject the sperm directly into the egg. In cases where the woman's menstrual cycles are irregular, or if she has scarring in her fallopian tubes, IVF frequently involves the use of hormones to help the ovaries with regular release of eggs, or sometimes to force the release of a number of eggs at once. In the latter case, eggs can be harvested and used for IVF, thus working around the scarring of the fallopian tubes.

The Roman Catholic Church prohibits most IVF techniques, especially those that involve the use of purchased sperm or eggs. Catholic theologians consider such use of a sperm or egg morally problematic for a couple of reasons: because an outsider has become involved in the act of reproduction, it is a form of adultery; and because sperm donation involves masturbation, it is an abuse of sexuality. They maintain that the use of IVF removes the natural connection between sexuality and reproduction. Most other denominations, however, have not taken as negative a stance toward IVF; nor have many churches prepared position papers on IVF, an indicator that they do not perceive it to be the sort of serious moral issue that, say, abortion is.

For a statement by the Christian Reformed Church on some of these life issues, see www.crcna.org/pages/positions_life.cfm.

But IVF and its related technologies do raise a number of ethical issues, and people with a number of different perspectives have raised concerns about the widespread use of ART. One of these concerns is the way ART may encourage parents to think of the children born as a result of these techniques as really theirs, suggesting, by implication, that adoptive children are somehow *not* really theirs. This implication is extremely problematic, especially in the context of purchasing sperm, eggs, or embryos, since the children produced in all of these cases are (genetically) no more their parents' "own" than adoptive children would be.

Many critics find the value system embedded in this sort of language and the attitudes perpetuated by those who offer ART unacceptable. The relationship of children to their parents is not determined by genetic connections—or the lack thereof. Any rhetoric that idolizes genetic ties is problematic. As Christians, we know that putting our ultimate hope of happiness in having biological children is really a bad idea. The danger of ART is that it may treat children as desirable (and expensive) products. So Christian parents who decide to use ART need to recognize and resist this aspect of the technology.

There are a variety of ways to maintain a different value system when using ART. Couples who go through infertility treatment frequently report that once they start, there is enormous pressure to continue trying over and over again. The church community can help by providing a space where people can talk about the responsible use of their resources—including money, time, and mental energy—in the pursuit of childbearing. We need to recognize that the desire to have children is good, but, like any desire, it can turn astray. Setting reasonable limits on resources to be spent and planning in advance can be of great help to people who want to resist those pressures.

Churches can also help keep the desire for children in perspective by making sure they create communities where the pressure to procreate is not overwhelming. Those who choose not to have children and those who cannot have children should experience the church as a welcoming place, not as a place where they feel like second-class citizens. Further, it should be possible for childless folk who enjoy children to participate in their lives on a regular basis, whether through formal or informal godparent relationships or through participation in church activities. When we take the perspective that the children of the church belong to the whole community, we make it possible to spread both the wonderful pleasures as well as some of the work of child-rearing around the community.

But pressure to procreate at whatever cost is not the only issue related to ART the Christian community needs to grapple with. Another is the changing nature of the relationship between parents and children. Purchasing sperm, eggs, or embryos in the course of infertility treatment is protected by medical confidentiality, as it should be. But that does not mean such issues cannot be discussed in the context of the church. The purchase of eggs or sperm cells, many have argued, represents a problematic shift in our thinking about having children. A child is a gift that comes to us in the context of the love of mother and father, sometimes expressed in their sexual unity, other times in their joint decision to adopt. But when a child is the product of purchased eggs or sperm, and when the characteristics of the individual selling the egg or sperm are examined by the purchaser to make sure they are acceptable, we have moved into a different sort of relationship to our children—and it is not clear that it is a healthy one.

> "To form a family ought not be an act of planning and control by which we replicate ourselves or gain access to a pleasurable experience of our own worth. It ought to be an act of faith and hope . . . ."
>
> —Gilbert Meilaender, *Body, Soul, and Bioethics*

Worries about how ART might change the relationship between parents and children in troublesome ways are, in some ways, hard to substantiate. But ART also raises specific concerns about the use of techniques that have not been adequately tested and are therefore potentially problematic. One is the use of hormonal stimulation to induce hyperovulation in women. Women have two ovaries, and in the normal course of things, each month one or the other ovary releases an egg that can potentially be fertilized. When doctors want to use IVF, they frequently induce hyperovulation—they use chemicals that mimic hormones to stimulate the ovaries to produce several eggs all at once. These eggs can then be harvested. Sometimes the same hormones are used to help a woman ovulate more regularly, or to produce more eggs when her partner's sperm are slower or sparser, in the hope that with more eggs, less mobile sperm will have a better chance of successfully fertilizing an egg.

The long-term effects of the chemicals used to stimulate hyperovulation on women's health are unknown. So we use them without knowing if they pose a health risk for women in general, or perhaps for women who have familial/genetic risk factors (a family history of ovarian cancer is one of the central concerns). Similarly, we simply don't know the long-term effects of achieving fertilization by injecting the sperm directly into the egg, but this technology is also widely used. We don't know whether sperm that have a hard time fusing with an egg might have other genetic abnormalities that could affect the child produced by this method.

Faced with this uncertainty, we ought not to assume, Chicken Little style, that the worst possible scenario is the truth. But the lack of adequate research on these issues does suggest that we may be rushing to use technologies before doing the careful work needed to find out whether they are safe for those involved in their use.

EMBRYO SELECTION AND THE PROBLEM OF UNWANTED EMBRYOS
One of the ironic side effects of using ART is that it may be *too* successful. Many couples who use IVF end up with a number of additional embryos. In some cases this is deliberate. For instance, couples who have a known family history of certain genetic diseases may choose IVF so they can screen the embryos for the disease and implant only those without the condition. In this case the embryos with the genetic condition will be discarded. Other couples may simply find that with hyperovulation they are able to generate eight or nine embryos, but they only want one or two children. When that happens, they need to decide what to do with the rest of the embryos they've produced.

This decision does not need to be made immediately. Embryos can be frozen (this is called *cryopreservation*); some of these embryos have been thawed and successfully implanted as much as twelve years after their initial generation. Nonetheless, parents need to take seriously their responsibility to decide what to do with their extra embryos.

Currently the options parents have are these:

▸ Discard excess embryos.
▸ Donate them for experimental use.
▸ Make them available through an infertility clinic.
▸ Make them available for adoption through an organization that facilitates adoption, such as Bethany Christian Services.

Many Christians find the first two options problematic, as both involve the destruction of the embryo. Bethany Christian Services (www.bethany.org) offers embryo adoption as one of its adoption possibilities. It is very careful to identify the procedure as a type of adoption. Parents who donate embryos provide basic family health histories and information for the adoptive parents and child. Infertility clinics, on the other hand, do not always consider donated embryos as a form of adoption. For the most part they refer to embryo donation as if it were on a par with other IVF techniques. This means that the children who are born as a result of this technology may have no knowledge of their genetic history.

THE COMMERCIALIZATION OF REPRODUCTION AND PREGNANCY

Finally, these technologies make it possible for people other than the parents—even complete strangers—to be involved in reproductive activities in a number of ways: by purchasing sperm anonymously over the Internet, for example. Or by purchasing embryos from infertility clinics who make them available along with their other services. In addition, the use of surrogate mothers who are willing to carry a baby to term for a fee has become so commonplace that you can find ads for these services in newspapers nationwide. Neither sperm donation nor surrogacy are completely new practices—the Old Testament leviratic law giving a widowed woman the right to have children with her husband's brother (most famously and disastrously broken in the case of Onan), as well as the story of Sarai and Hagar, indicate that similar procedures have been used since biblical times. But the advent of today's assisted reproductive technologies make it possible to reduce reproduction and pregnancy to a commodity available for purchase, a worrisome trend in which having children has become a potentially lucrative business.

> "As babies and children become products, mothers become producers, pregnant women the unskilled workers on a reproductive assembly line."
>
> —Barbara Katz Rothman, *Recreating Motherhood*

Both religious and secular thinkers hold one central moral rule: that is, humans ought not to be treated as objects to be used by others. In secular contexts, the phrase "human dignity" is often used to describe this concept, and it is a basic aspect of protection of human rights. The principle of autonomy, likewise, is intended, in part, to protect individual rights. Christians link the notion of human dignity with the doctrine that humans are made in the image of God, and so ought not to be treated in ways that are disrespectful of that image. Treating humans as if they were products that could be ranked in terms of their consumer value, or bought and sold on websites, seems to contradict this dignity and respect.

Buying sperm, eggs, or embryos, or hiring the services of a surrogate treats women and children as objects rather than imagebearers. Here again we see how the possibilities offered by technology can change human relationships—before ART, no parent ever had to decide whether or not to tell their child that she began as an embryo from an infertility clinic.

As we've mentioned, organizations that offer adoptive services for embryos, including Bethany Christian Services, are very clear that what they offer is embryo adoption, in contrast to some clinics that portray purchasing an embryo as somehow a matter of having "a real child of one's own." The former is a more honest way to frame the issue and is more respectful of the relationships involved. Embryo adoption, then, offers a way of approaching these issues with integrity. What about other types of commercial interventions—purchased sperm or egg, or commercial surrogacy?

It is harder to see how either of these could be used without making an object, to some degree, of someone in the relationship (sperm donor, surrogate, or child). When a sperm donor is selected purely on the basis of physical characteristics, or when a surrogate is asked to sign a contract stating that she will undergo amniocentesis and an abortion if the child has Down syndrome (a standard clause in surrogacy contracts), it is clear that both are being treated as an object to be used for someone else's purposes. Even the language we use for these exchanges indicates our discomfort with the commercialization involved: although people sell their sperm, we call them sperm "donors"—as if the relationship were that of a gift-giver and receiver.

GENETIC CONDITIONS

Many thinkers have noted this tendency for ART to turn the various parts of reproduction into commercialized relationships, and they also note the way that such commercialization harms the relationships between parents and children. But the commercial aspects of assisted reproductive technologies also raise a separate set of issues. When parents are paying large amounts of money for a child, there is a tendency to assume that only a perfect child will do. The story at the beginning illustrates that assumption—both Dr. Pascale and the Simons seem to accept the notion that an embryo with Down syndrome would not be a candidate for implantation.

Critics of ART argue that the use of these technologies encourages the assumption that only certain children are acceptable, an assumption that directly contradicts the Christian concept that all humans are God's image-bearers. Assisted reproductive technologies, these critics further argue, encourage us to consider some lives more valuable than others—and some simply not worthy of life at all.

This is a valid concern. At the same time we should be careful not to oversimplify the issue. When embryo selection is used to identify serious genetic defects, for example, we are in no position to condemn parents who choose to implant only embryos without those defects. It is easy for those who do not face such a choice to judge the actions of those who do. But if we would advocate for the implantation of embryos with serious genetic defects, we should also then help provide the resources families need to raise such children. In the absence of that support, condemnation of others' choices rings hollow.

We also need to recognize that that there are significant differences among the genetic conditions identified by testing that might give rise to concerns. Down syndrome, for example, a condition that is relatively easy to identify, causes a condition that is compatible with a full and satisfying life. Contrast that with Huntington's disease—Huntington's affects people between the ages of thirty-five and fifty; it causes a devastating degenerative condition that ends in death. There is no treatment and no reprieve. Other genetic conditions offer similarly bleak outlooks. Tay-Sachs disease, for example, affects the body's ability to metabolize certain lipids properly; it results in neural degeneration that produces blindness, deafness, and an inability to swallow. There is no treatment, and death is inevitable. Parents who choose not to implant embryos that test positive for any of these conditions do so because they believe they are incompatible with a decent life.

Most genetic conditions, on the other hand, are more ambiguous than Down syndrome or Huntington's disease. Most identifiable conditions involve a predisposition to develop particular symptoms, but only under certain conditions. There is a genetic sequence that predisposes some people to get schizophrenia, for example, but many of those who have the gene will not get the disease. (Even when identical twins have the gene and are raised in pretty much the same environment, there is only a 30 to 50 percent chance that if one twin has it, the other will as well.) There are a number of other genetically-linked conditions as well that indicate only that the child is at a higher risk for the condition, but not that she will get it. Similarly, because genetic sequence is only one risk factor, there are many people who do not have the gene in question who nonetheless end up with the condition.

Regardless of how we feel about these issues, the reality is that technology has given parents a new set of choices to make. Parents have the option of using assisted reproductive technologies that allow embryos to be created in vitro. They can have these embryos tested for a variety of genetic conditions. This reduces the chance of bringing into the world a child who will face severely destructive genetic conditions. On the other hand, it means parents will be tempted to consider any genetic abnormalities to be unacceptably risky.

As Christians formulate a response to these new technologies, we need to practice a number of virtues together. First, we must not heap burdens on another's back that we are not willing to bear ourselves. But we also need to resist the temptation to adopt the values of the world we live in. Our response should be colored by our belief that God's love is not limited to children and adults who are healthy, intelligent, and productive. God's banquet is spread out for the blind, the lame, and the poor—and those who think they have no need for a physician are likely to miss out on the celebration. Our calling is to love not only children who are "perfect," but all of God's children. Because all are made in God's image.

Questions for Reflection and Discussion

1. Assisted reproductive technologies are not cheap. In vitro fertilization and implantation costs about $10,000-12,000 for one attempt; the live birth success rate for one cycle, using fresh, non-donor eggs is around 30 percent. Should churches and fellow Christians help out with the financial burden as part of their ministry? Or should we be wary of these expenditures? Why?

2. In what ways can the church provide support (other than monetary) for couples who struggle with infertility?

3. Questions about embryo selection raise many of the same tough ethical questions that are raised with respect to abortion. How does the Christian belief that we are a community created in and living out a law of love for all of God's children shape our thinking about these questions?

For Further Reading

Ryan, Maura. Ethics and Economics of *Assisted Reproduction: The Cost of Longing*. Washington, D.C.: Georgetown University Press, 2001.

Waters, Brent. *Reproductive Technology: Towards a Theology of Procreative Stewardship*. Cleveland: Pilgrim Press, 2001.

Meilaender, Gilbert. *Body, Soul, and Bioethics*. Notre Dame: University of Notre Dame Press, 1995.

CHAPTER 8

Embryo Research and Cloning

S teve hangs up the phone. "You'll never guess who that was!" he says. "Congressman Black is working on legislation to ban cloning and stem cell research here in West Virginia, and he wants to run it past some citizen focus groups. He got my name from Pastor Chris at church—I guess because I work in biotechnology. But all I do is develop the results of genetic tests—I don't work with stem cells!"

"At least you're familiar with the subject," replies his wife, Maria. "That's worth something. And you must have opinions about whether stem cell research is OK or not."

"I'm conflicted," Steve replies. "I know some people think all stem cell research is wrong because it involves killing embryos. But I also know researchers hope that stem cells might offer a cure for Parkinson's—too late for my dad, but not for lots of other people. So I just don't know what to think."

"Maybe you need to just go and be confused, then," she responds. "It *is* a complicated issue—so there's nothing wrong with arguing for further study instead of a ban. And isn't that what focus groups are for, anyway? To talk these things through?"

"I'll at least think about it," says Steve. "I know I don't want anyone cloning people, anyway, so that part of the ban seems fine with me."

◆ ◆ ◆ ◆ ◆ ◆ ◆

Chapter 7 looked at the complexities of assisted reproduction—almost seeming to move, at times, into a brave new world of manufactured human beings. In this chapter we turn to the even more complex world of research involving embryos, stem cells, genetic manipulation, and cloning. These rapidly evolving technologies raise many of the issues we considered in our discussion of abortion and assisted reproduction. But they also raise important questions connected with chronic diseases such as Parkinson's and about how we allocate health care dollars.

One of the central issues raised by embryo research is that of public policy. Many argue that any such research should be banned. Others point out that such a ban conflicts with deeply held values of liberty and intellectual freedom to explore scientific questions. Still others argue that research has the potential to improve people's lives by offering new treatments for chronic conditions and various genetically linked diseases, so it is worth pursuing. Christian voices can be found on all sides in this debate. In this chapter we'll separate cloning from stem cell research and genetic manipulation; we'll consider what is at issue in each area, even though they are not completely separate. We'll begin with a brief overview of the technological wizardry involved with cloning, stem cells, and genetic manipulation.

> "Because of the intensity with which religious groups have struggled in the past over abortion, and because of the link between that debate and the question of the human embryo, intense religious conflicts over the status of the embryo and the legitimacy of embryo research have helped create a political stalemate. As a result, the federal government does not fund any embryo research, but it does not prevent it, either. Publicly funded researchers, who are held to high standards of public accountability, cannot conduct this work in the United States. Privately funded researchers, with almost no legal constraints, however, can pursue this work at will."
>
> —Ronald Cole-Turner, *God and the Embryo*

BASIC CONCEPTS

Human embryos are cells created when a human egg and sperm join through the process called fertilization. Previously, human embryos existed only inside women's bodies where they were largely impossible to see or study. But with the advent of in vitro fertilization (IVF) and related technologies, as well as extensive research on animal reproduction, scientists can now create, manipulate, and experiment on human embryos in the laboratory.

Cloning

Cloning is one of the techniques made possible by manipulation of embryos and gametes (see sidebar below). Although cloning refers to any procedure that produces two genetically identical individuals (technically, for example, identical twins are clones), the debate about the ethics of cloning refers specifically to somatic cell nuclear transfer (SCNT) technology, which for the rest of this chapter we'll simply call cloning. This is a technique whereby the DNA from the cell of one individual is put into the emptied nucleus of an egg cell from another individual. Egg cells only have half the normal number of chromosomes (the other half are provided by the sperm in a normal embryo). But the nucleus of any of an individual's cells has a full complement of DNA, and when this is inserted into the egg (and a variety of complicated techniques are used to initiate development) the egg can become an embryo—that is, a cell with a full set of chromosomes that is capable of developing into an individual.

> A gamete is a cell that fuses with another gamete during fertilization or conception. In humans, the female gamete is called an ovum or egg; the male gamete is called a sperm. Gametes carry half the genetic information of an individual, one chromosome of each type.

This technique was used to create Dolly, the famous cloned sheep. Since then, scientists have cloned a number of other mammals including dogs, cats, cows, and rabbits. In principle, cloning humans is possible, and various groups (some scientific, some not) have claimed to do so. But to date cloning has not been used to create a fully developed human baby genetically identical to the individual who provided his or her DNA. Genetic identity does not, of course, mean personal identity (as anyone who knows identical twins is aware), and a cloned individual would also have received some inherited material from the egg donor (RNA from the cellular material, for example). But cloning provides a method for obtaining an individual whose genetic makeup is mostly known in advance.

There is widespread international agreement that *reproductive cloning* (using the technology to create a baby) is morally unacceptable. Cloned embryos from other animals have a very low success rate for development, and some animals created from cloning have had serious health problems. Since we cannot ensure that cloning can be used safely, it should not be used for human reproduction. So the main debates about cloning these days concern the use of cloning technology for research and for the development of new therapeutic techniques. This is often called *therapeutic cloning* to distinguish it from reproductive cloning.

Stem Cells

In embryos that are allowed to develop for a short period of time, the cells divide repeatedly and eventually form a sphere called a *blastomere*. Within the central cavity of the blastomere are a number of cells—called *stem cells*—that will eventually go on to develop all the different tissues of the developing organism—some will become liver cells, others lung cells, skin cells, or the many other tissues that make up complex organisms. These stem cells are particularly valuable from a scientific standpoint because they are both *undifferentiated* (they aren't yet determined to be a particular kind of tissue) and *totipotent* (they have the capacity to become any of the different types of cells the body needs). Studying stem cells provides scientists with an understanding of the various developmental pathways different tissues follow. Understanding these pathways can lead to better treatments for cancers and genetic diseases, as well as techniques for slowing or reversing degenerative diseases.

Medical researchers are particularly interested in stem cells because their unique nature makes them suitable for specific types of cures. There is some evidence, for example, that it may be possible to use stem cells to help reconnect severed nerves for victims of spinal cord injuries. Scientists hope that properly prepared stem cells might have the potential to regenerate connections in the spinal cord and allow the individual to regain movement. Stem cells may also have the capacity to grow into insulin-producing cells for diabetics, or to help slow (or even stop) the progression of degenerative neurological disorders like Parkinson's disease. Finally, stem cells also have the potential to grow into particular organs. Sheets of cells that can be manipulated to develop into skin cells, for example, could be used to generate skin grafts for burn patients.

In addition to harvesting stem cells from embryos, scientists can retrieve stem cells from two additional sources: from the umbilical cord when a baby is born and from the bone marrow of adults. Some researchers argue that stem cells from these two sources are not as useful for research as embryonic stem cells; others argue that they are just as useful for research and therapeutic purposes. Until further research is done we simply don't know for sure.

The use of cloning together with stem cell manipulation is of particular interest for researchers who study organ transplant techniques. One of the central problems for transplanting organs is that the body's immune system reacts to a transplanted organ as a foreign intruder and tries to kill it. Immunosuppressant drugs are used to prevent this immune reaction, but they can have serious side effects that can cause other problems. But if an individual knew in advance that he would need a particular organ, it might some day be possible to create a cloned embryo from that person and use its stem cells to grow an organ for transplanting. This organ would be an almost perfect genetic match and thus would not cause antibody reactions.

Genetic Manipulation

The final technique we'll discuss in this chapter is *genetic manipulation*, a procedure that involves making changes in the DNA of an individual. Scientists know how to use virus-like entities to insert small chunks of genetic material into the DNA of a cell (though at this point they are not able to insert it in specific sites, so the application is limited). This has the potential to allow them to modify or even correct genetic defects in a developing embryo at very early stages. It may be possible to correct conditions involving the lack of the genetic sequences needed to generate certain proteins by manipulating the genetic material of the developing embryo. In this case the change in genetic makeup becomes part of the whole organism's genetic structure, and will be passed on to future generations if that individual has children. This is called *germ line gene therapy*. On the negative side, many scientists worry that tinkering with the complex structure of the genetic code without full understanding of how all the parts work together could pose future risks that have not yet been identified.

"The advent of cloning and other genetic technologies means that we human beings may soon be putting our hands on our own genetic endowment, in ways that will affect the humanity and identity of our children and our children's children. A novel responsibility is now upon us: to decide whether or not it is wise for us to grasp this awesome power over future generations, and if so, under what conditions and for what purposes."

—Leon Kass, *Human Cloning and Human Dignity*

Gene therapy is also being investigated for use in cases of fully-developed individuals. In this case the research is designed to create just a few cells of the desired type in an individual who lacks certain necessary genes. This type of manipulation, called *somatic cell genetic manipulation*, does not affect the sperm or eggs of the individual being treated and would not have an effect on any future children. It has been used experimentally to treat certain types of genetically linked auto-immune diseases in children, for example. Some of this research is quite promising, but it has also been problematic. One study in France was halted when a significant proportion of the children being treated for an immune disorder were found to have developed leukemia as a result of the therapy. In the United States, Jesse Gelsinger, a young man who suffered liver damage, died as the result of an experimental gene therapy technique, causing widespread concern about these techniques.

Finally, being able to identify and sometimes manipulate genetic sequences associated with various characteristics offers the future possibility of what some call "designer children." This refers to the ability of selecting or manipulating embryos to make sure the resulting child would have certain desirable characteristics. One rudimentary form of selection already occurs when parents undergoing IVF have their embryos screened for certain genetic defects before implantation. Embryos are sometimes also screened for sex, either because the parents simply prefer a child of a particular sex or because they have a sex-related genetic condition such as hemophilia. (The recessive gene for hemophilia is on the X chromosome. Since boys get only one X chromosome, from their mother, they have a 50 percent chance of having the gene that causes the disease if their mother is a carrier.)

Each of the three techniques we've described—cloning, stem cell research, and genetic manipulation—raises difficult moral issues. We'll take them one at a time, recognizing that there are commonalities among them.

ETHICAL ISSUES IN CLONING

As we've already mentioned, reproductive cloning is considered morally unacceptable (though it is not legally prohibited) worldwide. Any attempt to produce a child by cloning is likely to involve serious risk of harm to that child. Because it is universally recognized that subjecting a child to serious risk of harm in order to achieve a particular genetic identity is simply wrong, there is not much debate about reproductive cloning as things stand now.

In the future, as techniques get better and safety issues are resolved, the debate will most likely be reopened. We can expect to see questions arise about whether parents should be legally prohibited from cloning, or whether the free market in assisted reproductive technologies should extend to cloning. In addition to the safety considerations, from a Christian standpoint it is very difficult to endorse reproductive cloning. In the words of some authors, it represents an example of "parental narcissism"— those who seek a child for selfish, instrumental reasons.

Therapeutic cloning, however, offers a more complicated set of issues. It represents a very important set of potential therapies for a range of chronic and life-threatening conditions. Many scientists believe that this potential means we should endorse the use of cloning to create embryos for research and for stem cells in order to investigate these possibilities. Those who define embryos as fully human, on the other hand, reject therapeutic cloning because it involves the destruction of these embryos. There is currently no legal consensus on cloning at the national level in the United States, though a number of states have passed legislation. Some states ban reproductive cloning but not therapeutic cloning (California, Louisiana, and Rhode Island) while others ban both forms of cloning (Arkansas, Iowa, Michigan, and North Dakota). All of this legislation specifically targets cloning for the sake of stem cell research, research that has the greatest potential for producing medical benefits and economic profits in the relatively near future. It says very little about therapeutic cloning designed to generate new scientific information about processes of development.

STEM CELL CONTROVERSIES

On August 9, 2001, President George W. Bush announced a federal policy for the use of human embryonic stem cells in research. The policy limits the use of federal funds for such research to embryos created before that date, for reproductive purposes, and for which donors provided informed consent and received no financial incentives. The National Institutes of Health (NIH) notes that stem cells cultured from seventy-one different sources are available for this research. Critics have charged that only a very small portion of the seventy-one are suitable for research (some of the stem cell lines appear to have been contaminated by mouse DNA, others are not sufficiently viable for research purposes; for research to be adequate there must be enough different lines to ensure that any results are not idiosyncratic to the specific cells used). The policy prohibits only federal funding of any other sort of stem cell research, but not the research itself. Partially in response to this policy, Californian voters passed Proposition 71 in 2005, a measure that proposed to provide $3 billion in funding for embryonic stem cell research from state funds. Since that time, at least ten other states have considered similar programs (though none quite so large), spurred in part by a desire to improve their biotech business environment.

Although embryonic stem cells could be acquired after cloning, the vast majority available today for research come from embryos produced during attempts at assisted reproduction (so-called "spare embryos"). It is estimated that there are around 100,000 or more of these embryos frozen in various storage facilities, although many have been frozen for a number of years and are of limited viability. Most couples who undergo assisted reproduction do so because they want a child who is genetically related to them and the number of women who are willing to carry other people's embryos to term is small—thus the many excess embryos frozen in storage facilities.

> As we discussed in chapter 7, parents must decide what to do with their excess embryos: besides making them available for experimental use or making them available for sale in infertility clinics, they may choose to make them available for adoption through adoption agencies that provide this service. In this case, parents are asked to provide medical histories. See also page 84.

Stem cell research generates a long list of ethical questions:

- What is the status of an embryo that will never be implanted?
- Is it morally different from an embryo that will be implanted and may go through the process of development from which all of us originate?
- Do the potential benefits of stem cell research outweigh the moral costs of the destruction of embryos needed for this research?
- Does the consent of donors make the use of embryos acceptable?
- What sorts of research can be done on stem cells?

- Must the conditions studied in this research be serious disease conditions, or could cosmetic procedures be studied?
- Should any economic benefits that could be generated by stem cell research be thought of as belonging, in part, to the donors of the embryos used in the research?
- If stem cell research is undertaken with federal or state funding, should the profits from any resulting treatments belong to a pharmaceutical company?

The answer to most of these questions is connected to the answer one gives to the first and second questions: What is the status of an embryo that will never be implanted? If embryos, whatever their location or future potential, are defined as fully human beings, as they are by the official position of the Roman Catholic Church, then the answers to the rest of the questions become relatively straightforward. Since all stem cell research involves the destruction of the embryos used to generate stem cells, all such research is morally unacceptable. This approach is summed up by Charles Colson: "The whole idea of producing humans for body parts or for stem cells may sound appealing to some, but it will lead inevitably to the abolition of humankind and the ultimate end of Western civilization as we know it." Although this position offers a clear and uncompromising standard; it also puts its adherents in clear opposition to the trajectory of much of the modern world.

For those who do not identify embryos with full-blown humanity, the challenge is to specify the moral status of embryos and then to decide what that permits or prohibits. Both Christians and non-Christians alike argue that while embryos deserve a significant level of moral respect because of their potential to develop into humans, this potential is not morally equivalent to fully developed humanity. This view of embryos as morally significant (more than "just tissue") but not fully human (so that their use and destruction is not governed by, say, the laws governing human subject research) seems to allow as morally permissible their use in research on serious health problems, with the consent of those who donate them. Such use should never be taken lightly: adherents to this position might rule out scientific investigation into purely cosmetic procedures, for example, but otherwise place few restrictions on research.

Theologian Gene Outka argues that a middle-of-the-road position is preferable to either of these two extremes. He would permit research on embryos that have been created in the process of assisted reproduction but have no chance of being implanted and brought to term but prohibit the creation of embryos for the express purpose of research. He argues that since these embryos will perish whether they are used for research or not, using them for research is appropriate. At the same time, creating embryos expressly for research purposes (as is done in therapeutic cloning) represents too great a level of disrespect for the potential for human life that the embryo represents, and should therefore be banned.

Few theorists take up the thorny question of how economic matters are affected by these considerations. In general, United States courts have denied any claim to profits by individuals who contributed the tissues used in the development of various treatments. Legally, only the scientists who perform the research and the corporations who develop the commercial product are entitled to the profits of any pharmaceutical or treatment protocol.

Some argue that this legal assumption should be challenged: since embryos and stem cells represent the human biological potential that belongs to all humans, their use and the subsequent development of treatments should benefit the marginal and vulnerable in society, not just the large corporations that do the research. The history of the development of medicine suggests that this is unlikely to occur—the global poor have little access to high-tech medical procedures, even when the procedures in question develop, in part, from research on such populations. Typically the wealthy benefit the most from scientific research even though they are almost never research subjects.

GENETIC MANIPULATION AND "PLAYING GOD"

Running in the background of the stem cell debate is a very basic and difficult question. What sorts of manipulations and changes can we legitimately make to the human genetic code? Embryonic material intrigues scientists because it allows them to study the ways that single cells are able, in the right environment, and with the proper conditions, to almost magically move through a pattern of development that generates a far more complex organism than the cell that began the process. The normal course of things in the material world tends to be the exact opposite in terms of order—most organized systems have a tendency toward disorder and chaos, rather than increasingly complex organization. How is it that embryonic cells can move in the opposite direction?

These are issues scientists want to study. Many (though not all) of the answers to this question can be found in the genetic material the embryo contains, so the scientists' goal is to understand that material, manipulate it, and figure out what has gone wrong when it seems not to work. The hope is that when they are able to generate answers to these questions, they can use what they've learned to fix what seems to be wrong. In the same way that surgeons see a kidney transplant as a legitimate way of fixing one part of the body, scientists studying gene therapy hope to either replace or supplement defective genes with properly functioning ones that allow the body to function the way it should.

But while this analogy suggests that manipulating genes is no different from manipulating any other feature of the body, many worry that in manipulating the genetic code scientists are crossing an important moral line that perhaps ought not to be crossed. This question depends on two factors: First, what sort of manipulations do we envision? Second, what is it about the genetic code that makes it more worrisome than other manipulations?

> "There is grave uncertainty about our ability to say no and back-track when we detect abuses, especially if they have produced valuable scientific and therapeutic data or significant treatment. Medical technology . . . has a way of establishing irreversible dynamics."
>
> —Richard McCormick, "Should We Clone Humans?"
> *Ethical Issues in Human Cloning*

We raise the second question because the genetic code seems so central to our identity and thus to the nature of our very being. For those who identify embryos as complete human beings, the genetic material itself seems to signal humanity, and so any modification of that code seem to be the equivalent of tampering with the very self of the individual. For those who resist the definition of embryos as full human beings, on the other hand, modifications to the genetic code seem more on a par with other medical interventions.

Ironically, however, there is one form of genetic manipulation that causes the usual camps in bioethics to switch sides—when the genetic manipulation of the embryo before it has developed is used in order to correct or change particular genetic features—a process called germ line modification (see also p. 95). This kind of genetic manipulation changes the genetic code that an individual would pass on to any future children, so it could have an impact on many people. Because it is difficult to predict how genetic change would spread through a population, or what the long-term effects might be, many of the thinkers who are generally more willing to allow stem cell research would ban this particular sort of intervention. In somewhat surprising opposition to that position, the Roman Catholic Church would allow genetic manipulation of the embryo so long as it was performed for the good of the embryo. Their objection is not to genetic manipulation but to the use of the embryo for the benefit of others. Of course, this does not mean the church would unthinkingly endorse all manipulations, simply that they are more open to the possibility than many others.

CONCLUSION

These new technologies are fascinating, powerful, and worrisome. We need to wrestle with how they might fit into the life of the church and the Christian community. By focusing primarily on the wonderful things science has to offer, we can lose sight of the ways science can also contribute to inequalities and imbalances in the community. Our concern for the most vulnerable calls us in the Christian community to speak on their behalf—whether these are concerns about the vulnerable in our community being used as resources for other's benefit, or about the ways technologies can manipulate people and subject them to unacceptable risks so that pharmaceutical companies can increase their profits.

New genetic technologies and stem cell research seem to have great potential for curing or improving some devastating conditions. But the Christian community is one that embodies loving concern for the least among us. While we can embrace genetic technologies that also embody that concern, we should also be wary of the pressure exerted by new technologies to engage us in practices that are at odds with the story of Scripture.

Questions for Reflection and Discussion

1. In the story at the beginning of this chapter, Steve was asked to participate in a focus group on the subject of banning cloning and stem cell research. What position does your church have on this issue? Why? What would you say to Congressman Black if you were part of the focus group?

2. Genetic material is vitally important for the development of each individual into the person that she or he is. But many Christian thinkers argue that we should not be too quick to identify genes with identity. Allen Verhey argues that our identity is a matter of our relationship with God—we are created, loved children called to work in God's kingdom. Does this picture of identity strengthen or weaken the various arguments for or against genetic manipulation?

3. Individual Christians and various denominations disagree over the status of embryos and the moral acceptability of stem cell research. In spite of that disagreement we are called together to exemplify the unity of the body of Christ. In what ways can Christians who disagree on such matters find common ground for working together with other Christians?

For Further Reading

Colson, Charles and Nigel M. de S. Cameron, eds. *Human Dignity in the Biotech Century: A Christian Vision for Public Policy.* Downers Grove, Ill.: InterVarsity Press, 2004.

Mitchell, C. Ben, Edmund Pellegrino, Jean Bethke Elshtain, John F. Kilner, and Scott B. Rae, eds. *Biotechnology and the Human Good.* Washington, D.C.: Georgetown University Press, 2007.

Waters, Brent and Ronald Cole-Turner, eds. *God and the Embryo: Religious Voices on Stem Cells and Cloning.* Washington, D.C.: Georgetown University Press, 2003.

CHAPTER 9

GLOBAL HEALTH CARE

A n MSNBC story on January 29, 2008, focused on efforts of the poorest citizens of Haiti to feed themselves in the face of rising food costs and shortages. The solution these people had found was to eat mud—small patties or "cookies" made of mud, salt, and shortening. While eating mud staves off hunger for a while, eating it regularly causes malnutrition. But a "cookie" costs just five cents, while a bowl of rice (not exactly a balanced meal either) costs sixty cents. And the poor in Haiti are trying to survive on less than $2 a day.

Just over a month later, on March 2, 2008, Britain's *Independent* ran a news article about how much food gets thrown away in the United Kingdom—about twenty metric tons, a study determined, worth approximately £20 billion (roughly $35 billion). This wasted food, the story goes on to note, could meet half the food needs of Africa. It also points out that the United Kingdom is only one country among many developed nations. It may be more wasteful than other countries, but it is also a lot smaller. So it is likely that North Americans throw away far greater amounts of food.

These two stories highlight one of the most serious ethical problems in medicine—the problem of poverty and of global inequalities in health. We live in a world where millions of people face starvation and have almost no access to health care, while others throw away huge quantities of food and expect that thousands of dollars will be spent on their health care whenever they need it. The words of Mary's Song seem especially appropriate for those of us who live in the Western world: "He has scattered those who are proud in their inmost thoughts. He has brought down rulers from their thrones but has lifted up the humble. He has filled the hungry with good things but has sent the rich away empty" (Luke 1:51-53). And when we read Jesus' words in the parable of the sheep and goats, "Truly I tell you, whatever you did not do for one of the least of these, you did not do for me" (Matt. 25:45), it is hard for us to feel confident that we are not among the goats.

Up to now we've discussed bioethical questions that arise, for the most part, in the context of Western nations, including the United States, Canada, and the countries of the European Union, where good health care is widely available, though lack of access to insurance (in the United States) or immigrant status may make it hard for some to get good medical care. In much of the world, however, the problems are far deeper. These problems include lack of even the most basic medical treatments, poverty so severe that even simple treatments are too expensive for most people, and political instability that threatens to destroy even the minimal care that is available. It costs pennies to provide families in Africa with treated mosquito nets that can prevent malaria. But malaria is still rife in sub-Saharan Africa while we in American spend hundreds of thousands of dollars to provide a single person with a heart-lung transplant.

How should we address the disparities between the lives of those of us who live in wealthy nations and the world's poor? As Christians, we are called to extend our concern for others across national boundaries. When we see the suffering experienced by people living in some of the poorer nations in sub-Saharan Africa, especially when those who suffer are our brothers and sisters in Christ, we cannot turn away and pretend not to notice. In this chapter we'll examine the general questions raised by global inequalities of wealth and of access to basic health care. We'll look at some of the central Christian responses to these issues and examine how the rapid globalization of economic structures affects our response for good and for ill.

GLOBAL DISPARITIES IN HEALTH AND LIFE SPAN

We'll start with some basic facts from the World Health Organization (WHO), which provides extensive statistics about health issues worldwide, and then consider some of the factors that have generated the global system we inhabit.

The two factors that are generally used to measure health are mortality and morbidity. *Mortality* refers to the average life expectancy at birth: how long do people generally live, and at what ages are they at greatest risk of dying? *Morbidity* refers to the incidence of diseases of various sorts in the population: HIV/AIDS, tuberculosis, diabetes, cardiovascular disease, and the like. The two numbers are clearly related, but for purposes of understanding global health trends it is important to track both.

Developed countries with high rates of HIV infection and universal health care have lower mortality rates than countries where health care is not affordable for large numbers of the population, for example.

There is a huge gap in life span between wealthy nations like the United States and Canada and poorer nations, and the gap grows larger in countries that struggle with a combination of poverty, political instability, and human rights violations. Women in sub-Saharan Africa have a one in thirteen chance of dying in childbirth; in the developed world women have only a one in 4,085 chance. Life spans have remained stable or increased in the developed world—Japan currently has the highest at eighty-three years, closely followed by North America and Western Europe with rates that run around eighty. This contrasts sharply with countries that are torn apart by war (for people in Afghanistan, life expectancy in 2006 was forty-two years) or are dealing with devastating poverty or both. The lowest numbers are generally found in sub-Saharan Africa, where life expectancies range from the mid-forties to the mid-fifties. Even more disheartening, while life expectancies increased or remained the same throughout most of the world between 2000 and 2006, they decreased in several African nations (Lesotho, Ghana, and Gabon, for example).

> "The biggest enemy of health in the developing world is poverty."
> —Kofi Annan, former Secretary-General of the United Nations

While poverty alone does not cause poor health, there is a clear and uncontroversial connection between poverty and health problems. Countries with lower life expectancies and higher rates of infant mortality are all much poorer than those with higher life expectancies. This is not surprising. First, lack of money makes it hard for people to pay for basic necessities, much less expensive medical treatments. Second, poor countries have fewer government resources for providing even basic necessities such as clean water or immunizations, let alone hospitals and clinics or medical equipment. And third, because doctors and nurses in developing countries are paid so little compared to those in wealthy countries, there is an enormous "brain drain"—that is, the migration of trained medical workers out of poor countries into wealthier ones. In 2005 the BBC reported that 75 percent of Zimbabwean doctors trained in Zimbabwean medical schools had emigrated; the number of doctors trained in Ghana but registered to practice in the UK doubled between 1999 and 2004. This is particularly problematic because these countries are subsidizing medical education in an attempt to address the doctor shortage they face. When the doctors leave for greener pastures, the end result is that poor countries are subsidizing the health care of wealthier countries by supplying them with a (relatively) cheap supply of doctors.

But poverty alone accounts for only some of the differences in health around the globe. Countries with similar economic standing often have very different health data, and these data tend to diverge more sharply over time. Analysts have noted that levels of inequality in a country are almost as important as levels of poverty in predicting health disparities. For example, South Korea, a society with low levels of inequality, has achieved far greater reductions in both mortality and morbidity than Brazil, a deeply unequal society. In countries with lower levels of inequality, increasing the overall national wealth results in more health care for the poor; in countries with deep inequalities, increases in overall wealth merely widen the disparity between the wealthy and the poor.

Other factors that interact with poverty to make people's lives worse yet include political corruption, political instability, and violence. War and civil strife cause health problems in populations both because of the violence people suffer and because of the destruction of infrastructure (health clinics, housing, roads) that usually accompanies violence.

The statistics paint a clear overall picture: people who live in countries with stable political systems, high levels of wealth, and relatively equal distribution of wealth enjoy the lowest levels of mortality and morbidity, the highest life expectancies, and the lowest rates of infant mortality. Those who live in countries with unstable and corrupt political systems, high inequality, and low levels of overall wealth suffer the lowest life expectancies, the highest rates of infant mortality, and high rates of morbidity.

RESPONSES TO THE GLOBAL SITUATION

The global community has not been completely indifferent to this suffering. Over the years, a broad spectrum of institutions have attempted to respond to the suffering of the world's poor—with mixed results. The reasons for these mixed results are complicated. In some cases, success in one health initiative (childhood immunization, for example) can lead to other health issues (population growth, for example, contributes to the spread of infectious diseases). In other cases, health initiatives are undermined by war and ethnic cleansing. Some health initiatives fail because they are not financially sustainable, while others are undermined by various financial policies chosen by national governments or imposed by international financial organizations.

The World Health Organization (WHO), formed in 1948, addresses global health issues. It is the public health wing of the United Nations and plays a vital role in setting international health goals, providing accurate information about global health trends, and coordinating efforts to provide basic health care to the citizens of member states. It has enormous potential for good: its efforts to eradicate some of the devastating diseases that affect people worldwide (smallpox, polio, and other less well-known diseases such as trypanosomiasis, Guinea worm, dengue fever, and leprosy) have improved people's lives and health in vital ways. At the same time, as a subsidiary institution of the United Nations, the WHO has some of the same problems: a bloated bureaucracy and a tendency toward corruption. Its very size tends to make efficient action difficult. And the only punitive measure is has to deal with corrupt government officials (who often siphon away funds meant for public health) is international opinion.

Finally, the WHO cannot force donor nations to pay the amount they have pledged to address the needs of global health. In 2000, for example, leaders of 189 countries agreed on a series of eight "Millennium Development Goals," some of which impact health. The target date for meeting these goals is 2015. Unfortunately the first accounting in 2005 showed that most countries are off track for most of the goals, and some actually moved backward. The chief reason cited for the lack of progress on these goals was a lack of donor support. For example, to pay its share in 2004 the United States would have had to spend $75 billion rather than the $15 billion it actually provided. Measured by percentage of gross domestic product, the United States is among the stingiest of the developed nations in terms of supporting these initiatives. Denmark ranks first in the world, donating 1 percent its gross domestic product to foreign aid. The United States donated its highest percentage (0.58 percent) in the 1960s; since then it has donated smaller amounts (to a low of 0.11 percent in 2001, with small increases since then).

There's an old stand-up comic routine that calls to mind some of the issues of international aid: One character complains about a restaurant because the food's so bad; the second chimes in, "And the portions were so small!" We've already noted that there is not enough international funding to address many of the world's needs. Unfortunately the funding that is available is often used ineffectively, and sometimes even makes things worse. For example, in recent years most of the international food and development aid overall is used to purchase United States products or services, a policy economists call "tied aid." Requiring that services and food be purchased from United States suppliers has the effect of undermining local industries and is an inefficient way of providing services, but it is very popular with the American business community.

Add to this the tendency of the United States (and many other countries) to direct aid to strategic allies rather than to the neediest countries and to designate much of that aid for debt relief rather than actual relief programs, and it's not difficult to understand that the amount of money we spend on providing for actual health care needs of the world's poorest citizens is vanishingly small.

Over the last fifty years, other avenues have been established to provide for the needs of the world's poor. These include thousands of nongovernmental organizations (NGOs) that address a variety of global health issues. Some of these organizations are huge—the International Commission of the Red Cross, for example, is made up of almost 97 million volunteers, supporters, and staff; others are tiny. Some have been operating for almost ninety years (again, the Red Cross); others exist for only short periods of time. Together they have become a significant force for focusing global attention on health problems and responding to them in a timely fashion. In addition private foundations such as the Bill and Melinda Gates Foundation provide significant funding for improving health and reducing poverty in developing countries.

Unlike the World Health Organization, which has the very general mission of protecting and promoting health globally, NGOs and foundations generally have a very specific mission. The Red Cross, for example, was formed to provide medical assistance to the wounded (civilian and combatants) during war times. Over the years its mission has expanded to promoting humanitarian values, disaster response, disaster preparedness, and health and community care—a mandate that is almost as broad as that of the WHO. Médecins Sans Frontières (MSF, or Doctors Without Borders), an alternative medical assistance group, provides emergency medical assistance to populations in danger. While the Red Cross adopts a position of strict political neutrality, impartiality, and confidentiality, MSF deliberately adopts an attitude of advocacy. These organizations thus play very different roles on the international scene, and this has led to some tension between them. Because of its strict neutrality, the Red Cross has often been able to gain access to prison camps where the MSF is not allowed. This neutrality can be a double-edged sword, however. MSF members have accused the Red Cross of complicity in cases such as the ethnic cleansing that went on in the former Yugoslavia.

The tensions between the Red Cross and the MSF represent the strengths and weaknesses of most NGOs. Their specific mission allows them to engage in some activities and prevents them from engaging in others; this limited focus can be a weakness under certain circumstances. In the past, most health-related NGOs focused on specific health care issues (eye surgery, immunization, and the like). But because of the close connections between political structures, poverty, and health, more and more health-related NGOs have had to adopt specific political agendas, whether defending basic human rights (as in the case of Physicians for Human Rights, founded in 1986) or lobbying governments for equity for ethnic minority groups. Some NGOs are secular; others are explicitly religious. Both types are supported by individual Christians and by Christian organizations.

The work of NGOs complements the work of the World Health Organization but cannot substitute for it. Most NGOs can only address specific issues in particular areas, resulting in a piecemeal approach that fails to address many serious global health issues. And since NGOs remain in existence only as long as they can find funding, they are sometimes unable to offer sustained responses to global problems.

Most Christians are probably familiar with some of the Christian NGOs that address specific health issues worldwide. An organization called Christian Connections for International Health (CCIH) is one among a variety of networks designed to help Christian NGOs work productively, partner with other international health organizations, and design effective interventions for specific health issues. Numerous other organizations, including the Christian Reformed Church World Relief Committee, focus on alleviating poverty and assisting development and provide either emergency or long-term health care as part of their antipoverty efforts. And a wide variety of other Christian NGOs focus on various health issues around the world.

A complete survey of these organizations is beyond the scope of this discussion. But even this brief survey of organizations involved in public health work around the world puts us in a better position to think about the elements of an appropriate Christian response to global health issues.

CHRISTIAN RESPONSES

As members of the Christian community, Scripture calls us to respond to the needs of the poor. The question we face is *how* we should respond. Providing medical care of one sort or another has been an integral part of Christian mission work since the early days of the church, but we live in a world where medical resources are far more effective and far more wide-ranging than ever before—as well as far more expensive. We live in a world where the needs of the global poor are overwhelming and the difficulties in providing for them are enormous.

Christians in the United States have responded to the health needs of the world's poorest people in a variety of ways. Because many American Christians have adopted a relatively individualistic theology and belong to churches that are unaffiliated with larger denominations, the tendency is for churches to develop their own individual mission projects. This may take the form of individual mission trips by congregation members or raising funds for a particular project. These attempts are well-intentioned but not always especially effective. Individual mission trips generally do not result in long-term, sustainable change. In some cases those on the receiving end are no better off than they were before the mission appeared.

Short term mission trips go wrong when they appear to be
- Self-serving: provide value for visitors without meeting the local community's needs.
- Raising unmet expectations: send volunteers practitioners and trainees who do not have appropriate language or medical training or accountability.
- Ineffective: provide temporary, short-term therapies that fail to address the root causes.
- Imposing burdens on local health facilities: provide culturally irrelevant or disparaging care and leave behind medical waste.
- Inappropriate: fail to follow current standards of health care delivery (continuity, access) or public health programs (equity, sustainability).

—Parminder Suchdev, "A Model for Sustainable
Short-Term International Medical Trips"

Denominational groups and established mission programs are often better positioned to have a long-term impact on specific needs because they have the structural resources to provide sustained assistance. They can develop partnerships with those they intend to help that lead to a better understanding of needs and cultural and social circumstances. In order to be effective, development and health care assistance must be perceived by those who receive it as responding to their needs, and it has to be integrated into their lives. Further, it needs to be ongoing and to have built-in mechanisms to evaluate both its effectiveness at meeting goals and the appropriateness of the goals themselves.

Organizations such as the Christian Reformed World Relief Committee and World Vision are exemplary in this regard. They have a long history of identifying specific issues that have clear and measurable health benefits and establishing partnerships with community members to work on sustainable, long-term development projects. In Ghana, for example, World Vision works with local communities to develop boreholes—wells from which water can be pumped. These boreholes replace the contaminated rivers and pools that communities often use for their source of water. Open water is infested with Guinea worm, a horrible parasite that can cause paralysis and death. Before beginning a project, they involve the community in education about the causes of various waterborne diseases, enlist community members in the construction and maintenance of the borehole, and follow up to make sure that the well is maintained and used properly.

Development projects such as these can make huge long-term differences in people's lives. The availability of clean, safe water helps people avoid illness, and, in the case of women in rural Africa, also frees them from having to carry heavy barrels of water long distances every day, an exhausting and time-consuming task. These development projects directly improve people's health and lives and continue to provide benefits for years into the future.

NGOs, then, can make a difference in the lives of particular communities. But the huge disparities around the globe require a more systemic response than individual organizations can offer. In chapter 1 we discussed how Christian theology allows us to recognize the powers of this world—the large-scale societal forces that take on a life of their own and determine major aspects of people's lives. The global economy is certainly such a power. Global economic structures have established a world in which most of us reading this book can expect to live into our eighties and watch our children and grandchildren grow up healthy and strong. On the other side of the globe, people struggle to survive into their forties and watch children and grandchildren die of easily treated conditions. Those people are our sisters and brothers in Christ. Their sorrows over dying children, their short and difficult lives, must be our sorrows as well, for we are all members of the same kingdom of God.

The power of large-scale economic systems cannot be changed or challenged by individual actions. But it can be confronted by the worldwide church. As Christians we need to learn from our brothers and sisters in developing nations. We need to find out what forces prevent them from achieving decent lives, learn from their courage in confronting daunting challenges, and discover how to respond together in ways that respect the basic rights of all people. The Roman Catholic Church has been a leader in this regard, issuing pastoral letters on poverty that challenge all of us to recognize the importance of this issue for Christians. Imagine how God could work through the worldwide church if we could begin to speak with one voice, guided by the Holy Spirit, to challenge the economic structures that are so destructive of people's lives and health around the globe!

Questions for Reflection and Discussion

1. What is the relationship between poverty and health? What are some of the other issues that intersect with poverty to affect global health care?

2. Although poverty, disease, and political instability characterize much of the developing world, the vitality and growth of the Christian church in those areas far outstrips its presence in the developed world. Why do you think this might be? How can Christians in the developed world learn from the church in other countries about the church's mission?

3. Given that many Christians worldwide have no access to even basic health care, how should we evaluate the enormous expenditures most of us will eventually make on end-of-life care? How might we rethink our priorities in light of global inequalities?

4. Research some of the organizations you know of that address issues of global health care. Perhaps your denomination has one. (You may want to check out CRWRC, World Vision, Reformed Church World Service, and others.) What are they doing well? How can these organizations be part of the response of the worldwide church?

For Further Reading

Farmer, Paul. *Pathologies of Power: Health, Human Rights, and the New War on the Poor.* Berkeley, Calif.: University of California Press, 2005.

O'Neil, Edward, Jr. *Awakening Hippocrates: A Primer on Health, Poverty, and Global Service.* Chicago: American Medical Association Press, 2006.

Schlossberg, Herbert, Pierre Berthoud, Clark H. Pinnock, and Marvin Olasky. *Freedom, Justice, and Hope: Toward a Strategy for the Poor and Oppressed.* Westchester, Ill.: Crossway Books, 1988.

Van Til, Kent A. *Less Than 2 Dollars a Day: A Christian View of Poverty and the Free Market.* Grand Rapids, Mich.: Eerdmans, 2007.

CHAPTER 10

THE GLOBAL CHALLENGE OF HIV/AIDS

Covenant Redeemer Church is facing a unique challenge. The refugee family they're planning to sponsor—the Akols, a mother and her three children from the Sudan—are dealing with HIV. Miriam, the mother, and her youngest daughter, Sarai, are both HIV positive. The church has already sponsored several refugee families, but none with this health issue. It leads to spirited discussion in the council room.

"We've worked with people with a wide variety of health conditions before," points out Pastor Donaldson. "The Hmong family we sponsored in the eighties had two members with tuberculosis, which is more contagious than AIDS. HIV is no different, in my book."

"I wasn't here in the eighties," says Jeri, chair of the deacons. "But we have to deal with this as a congregation. People are scared of AIDS—we can't keep this information from the congregation. Besides, when they're helping with the baby they need to know enough to be careful about bodily fluids."

Another deacon shifts uncomfortably in his seat. "I hate to even bring this up," he says, "but can we afford to sponsor someone with AIDS? Immigrants aren't eligible for health care from Medicaid until they've been here for five years. I know Miriam is only HIV positive and doesn't have AIDS yet, but we don't know when she might start needing extensive medical care. What is our responsibility if she gets sick or if the baby gets sick?"

"I'm sure we can work something out with Social Services," Pastor Donaldson responds, hoping this is true. "But we do need to figure out this issue of informing people. Is this something we need to keep confidential, or should volunteers know about it?"

♦ ♦ ♦ ♦ ♦ ♦ ♦

In the previous chapter we looked at the issue of global health and at a few of the organizations that respond to the world's needs. In this chapter we focus on one of the largest global health crises in history: HIV/AIDS.

The church has been a vital part of the worldwide response to this crisis. In this chapter we look at why AIDS is such a problem and at how the church has addressed it in positive and negative ways.

A BRIEF HISTORY

The set of symptoms that characterize AIDS (acquired immunodeficiency syndrome) was first identified in the 1980s. Medical historians believe that the retrovirus that causes AIDS, the human immunodeficiency virus (HIV), had existed at low levels since at least the 1950s, probably originating in western equatorial Africa. But because AIDS occurred so sporadically and doctors had not yet linked the symptoms to a single disorder, it was not until several decades later that the syndrome was recognized and the virus identified. HIV/AIDS is particularly difficult to deal with because it has a very long incubation period, averaging nine years, during which the virus and the body's immune system battle for dominance. During this period the disease can be transmitted through body fluids (blood, genital fluids, or breast milk), though the infected individual will show few symptoms. About nine or ten years after infection, the immune system is so weakened that the symptoms of full-blown AIDS appear, and without treatment death usually follows in less than a year.

> "HIV/AIDS does not kill but destroys the immune system's capacity to resist other opportunistic infections that are ultimately fatal."
>
> —John Iliffe, *The African AIDS Epidemic*

Because HIV is a retrovirus, a very simple strand of RNA (rather than DNA) that mutates very quickly, it took some time to find effective medical responses. Researchers attempted a number of different treatments before discovering the current antiretroviral regimen that can keep the disease in remission for decades. Although there is no cure for the disease, it can be managed.

Antiretroviral drugs are expensive, and they must be taken at specific times on a regular basis. If these drugs are not taken regularly, the virus can begin to mutate and become drug resistant, posing a real danger of reviving the AIDS epidemic that threatened the world in the 1980s and 90s. For a number of years, the antiviral drugs that keep the disease under control were not available in the developing world. In addition to the high cost, public health workers argued that people who were poor and uneducated would be unable to maintain the complicated regimen of pill-taking. As a result of these two factors, AIDS continued to be a death sentence in poorer countries while becoming a manageable condition in the developed world.

From a moral standpoint, this situation demanded action. To address the first problem (the high cost of antiretroviral drugs), in recent years the world community has pressured pharmaceutical companies to produce cheaper generic versions of these antiretrovirals for distribution in the developing world. And since the populations most affected by HIV could not afford the high-priced versions of the drugs in any case, allowing low-cost generics to be sold in developing countries certainly has not hurt the profitability of drug companies.

Second, medical workers in developing countries have set up methods of providing the drugs on a carefully organized schedule and are educating people to take them appropriately. Research shows that the failure rate of taking antiretroviral drugs appropriately is not much higher in the developing world than in wealthier countries. The main issue continues to be expense: in countries where significant numbers of the population are trying to survive on less than two dollars a day, even generic, publicly financed antiretrovirals are out of reach of many who need them. And recent increases in the costs of fuel and food mean the world's poor find themselves even less able to gain access to these and other medicines.

There are other significant differences between the trajectory of HIV/AIDS in the developed world and the developing world. In Europe and North America, HIV/AIDS was initially a disease predominantly occurring in gay men and intravenous drug users—both populations that are relatively contained. Public health workers in those countries thus had relatively small, identifiable populations, extensive public funding, and stable political systems within which to work. They were able to make an impact on transmission rates relatively quickly (though recent years have seen a slight increase in transmission rates and in heterosexual transmission). Because most of the research on HIV/AIDS was conducted in Europe and the United States, HIV was perceived as a disease related to homosexuality, a perception that remains fairly prevalent throughout the world.

In Africa, public health workers face a disease that is spread out among the population generally and is exacerbated by the high mobility that poverty often generates. In sub-Saharan African, in particular, AIDS is passed on primarily either by heterosexual contact or by an infected pregnant woman to her baby during the birth process or while breast feeding. This occurs in societies with high levels of inequality (especially gender inequality) and low levels of education, where civil war and political unrest displace large numbers of people on a regular basis, and where the resources available for responding to health problems are heavily limited.

These demographic features make HIV/AIDS difficult to address. But social perceptions make it even more difficult to respond to the disease. The connection of HIV/AIDS with homosexuality has created a stigma that makes it much more difficult to study and treat in the African context, especially in countries with large Muslim populations. The combination of poverty and this stigma have made testing rates for HIV status very low. As a result, the virus continues to be passed on during its incubation period. In many African countries men refuse to use condoms and women do not have the social standing to demand that men use protection. Further, many government leaders believe that Western research into HIV/AIDS is racist. Some have argued that HIV is not the cause of AIDS and have resisted the use of Western medicines. This combination of factors has resulted in HIV infection rates that represent a global public health crisis.

Rates of HIV infection have declined slightly in the past year, but remain high in many countries in Southern Africa. In countries with the highest rates, such as South Africa and Botswana, as many as 20 percent of adults between the ages of fifteen and forty-nine are infected with the virus (the rate of infection in that age group in the United States is 0.6 percent). This is a devastating situation, because every country needs a relatively healthy adult population to maintain its economy and to raise and educate the next generation. High rates of HIV infection results in the phenomenon of AIDS orphans—children left parentless because of AIDS—and place serious pressure on health care systems that are already weak. Other African countries have lower rates of HIV infection (Angola and Nigeria, 3.7 percent; Kenya 6.8

"The global pandemic of HIV/AIDS remains the most important infectious disease threat to human health of our time. At this writing (mid-2005) perhaps 40 million men, women, and children are living with HIV infection and more than 25 million people have already died. In 2004, the world saw 5 million people become newly infected, underscoring the undone work of prevention, and 3 million deaths, stark evidence of our ongoing failure to provide treatment and care to the many millions who need it."

—Jonathan Cohen, Nancy Kass, and Chris Beyrer, "Human Rights and Public Health Ethics," *Public Health and Human Rights* percent) but even these lower rates represent a serious health challenge. AIDS is considered the most serious public health crisis facing the world today.

ETHICAL ISSUES RAISED BY HIV/AIDS

The first set of ethical questions raised by HIV/AIDS concerns individual rights issues such as mandatory testing and confidentiality. This is probably a reflection of AIDS in the developed world, since in that context, with localized populations of gay men and intravenous drug users at greatest risk of contracting HIV, people could make clear behavior choices to reduce their risk of contracting the disease. (For the thousands of hemophiliacs infected by blood transfusions, there were no behavioral safety precautions available, and there were many individuals in the early 1980s who lacked the ability to protect themselves.) But as researchers' understanding of the disease developed and public health safeguards such as testing blood donations became standard, avoiding HIV infection in the Western world has become relatively straightforward.

Initially mandatory testing was quite controversial: before there was effective treatment for the disease, testing did not clearly benefit the individual tested. And regardless of people's HIV status, their sexual partners could (presumably) choose safer sexual practices. Thus many in the West considered mandatory testing to be an unacceptable infringement of individual rights. Likewise, maintaining confidentiality about a person's HIV status fit well with Western medical practice.

In the African setting, the situation was quite different. As we've seen, instead of being limited to particular, high-risk demographics, rates of HIV infection were instead spread throughout the population. Women who were rarely in a position to refuse sex or demand safe sex practices were often blamed for HIV infections even when their male partners were more likely to have brought the virus home. In this context, the Western emphasis on protecting confidentiality and on protecting individuals from mandatory testing proved to be less appropriate. Health care workers often refused to provide care for anyone suspected of having AIDS—and, given the conditions under which health care delivery functions in much of Africa, their worries about contracting HIV were not entirely unjustified. Further, the community- and family-based systems of care that have characterized many African societies for centuries were not compatible with the individualistic model of confidentiality of Western medicine.

In some African communities, church-based groups have endorsed HIV testing before marriage; they discourage the marriage of those found to be

HIV positive. It is unclear whether this more communal response to HIV will turn out to be an effective method of slowing the rate of infection. In general, it seems clear that the ethical concerns that framed HIV/AIDS in the West need to revised in the context of other cultures. Similarly, responses to HIV/AIDS need to be adapted to specific cultural practices and context.

International aid agencies often set up HIV/AIDS intervention programs modeled on Western medical practice. This mindset produced a tendency to ignore the prevalence of HIV infection among women and children in Africa. Because HIV/AIDS in the West tends to be concentrated in male populations, it took several years of activism on the part of international women's groups before antiretroviral drugs were tested in women and before reducing maternal-infant transmission during and after birth became a priority. For example, the use of a drug called Nevirapine has been shown to reduce maternal transmission significantly and at a relatively low cost, and the savings it represents in terms of decreased medical expenses for babies makes it extremely cost-effective. But its use in African clinics was delayed, in part, by a lack of testing and a general focus on HIV/AIDS transmission among men.

The initial association of HIV/AIDS in the West with homosexual activity and drug abuse also contributed to a general stigma attached to positive HIV status. This stigma interacted with a general tendency for a moralistic response to disease. Such a response tends to frame the disease as a punishment by God directed toward specific sins. Those who believe that the sick person is responsible for bringing God's wrath on him- or herself have justified a response of repudiation, rejection, and shame. This moralistic response to HIV/AIDS has been common both in Africa and in North America, but in both contexts it has diminished with time. Most people now recognize that moralistic responses make it much harder for HIV positive individuals to admit their status or seek access to care.

Further, the shaming and ostracism that accompany a moralistic response are often misdirected. We've already noted that in some African countries it is common for HIV/AIDS to be transmitted by a husband who has engaged in extramarital sex to his wife. Because of the inequality of their status, women do not have any safe way of requiring their husband to use a condom. At the same time, the husband may blame the woman for being HIV positive and drive her out of the house, sometimes with their children. Or the husband's family might take the house and all the family's property after the husband's death, blaming his widow for bringing AIDS into the village.

> "The majority of married women who have [AIDS] have had no other partner than their husbands."
>
> —Nafis Sadik, Special Envoy of the United Nations Secretary-General for HIV/AIDS in Asia

Of course, this response is not unique to the African context. In 1984 a young American boy named Ryan White was diagnosed with AIDS, which he contracted from tainted blood transfusions. His community reacted with fear and discrimination when he expressed his wish to continue attending school and to live as normally as possible. Eventually he and his family moved to another community, where he attended school until his death in 1990. The case attracted national attention and exposed the fear and ignorance with which people treated those with HIV/AIDS at the beginning of the AIDS crisis, regardless of whether they contracted it through blood transfusions or homosexual contact.

Because moralistic responses have generated this sort of obvious injustice and cruelty, most advocates for HIV/AIDS prevention argue that a nonjudgmental, educational approach is preferable to a moralistic response. People need information about HIV transmission, testing needs to be easily accessible and confidential, and the general population needs extensive education about the causes of AIDS. More controversially, many HIV prevention programs advocate the use of condoms in what's called the "ABC" educational program: **a**bstain; **b**e faithful; use a **c**ondom.

The Roman Catholic Church has been very critical of this advocacy of condom use because of its longstanding condemnation of birth control. Catholic health care workers who focus on AIDS treatment and prevention in a variety of contexts thus find themselves in a difficult position. Although condom use is an effective component in HIV prevention, Catholic health care workers who advocate it risk being censured or even losing their jobs because of conflict with the church's theology. Worse, even though the church has accepted the legitimacy of a married couple's use of condoms to prevent transmission of HIV when one partner is positive, some Catholic health care workers tell women that they may not require their husbands to use condoms, on pain of God's punishment. At the same time, we should also recognize that the Roman Catholic Church worldwide has been a central leader in speaking out against the stigmatization of individuals with AIDS, providing care for the sick and dying, and focusing worldwide attention on the injustice of a global health system where the poor have no access to needed treatments.

One of the essential contributions of Christian theologians in the discussion surrounding HIV/AIDS is to shift from a narrow focus on individual sexual behavior to focusing on the social and gender issues that contribute to the worldwide spread of AIDS. As we've seen, poverty correlates closely with susceptibility to HIV infection, and global responses to poverty have frequently exacerbated the problem. In the 1990s, countries with large amounts of foreign debt were required to undergo structural adjustment programs designed to move their economies toward a free market model. Although these policies were based on what was then considered to be the best economic model available for improving the population's living conditions, they actually had the effect of requiring countries to cut the already small amounts of government funding provided for health care and basic needs such as clean water. This withdrawal of public funds from health care exacerbated the health problems caused by HIV/AIDS.

Because the HIV/AIDS crisis is connected with social structures and poverty, it is not surprising that a central debate in the global discussion about HIV/AIDS concerns economics. Two questions have been particularly difficult:

▸ First, what percentage of available funds should be used for treatment versus prevention of HIV/AIDS?
▸ Second, how much international aid funding should be directed toward AIDS versus other diseases, particularly malaria and tuberculosis?

Some theorists argue that those already infected are the sickest and most in need of care; others argue that prevention is more cost effective than treatment. In Africa, AIDS has surpassed both malaria and tuberculosis as the leading cause of death. It is a serious health problem in the developed world as well. Since 1990 AIDS has been the leading cause of death of black men in the United States between the ages of thirty-five and forty-four, and the second leading cause of death among black men and women between the ages of twenty-six and thirty-six. It is clear that the world needs to respond to the disease with significant resources. But funds available for health care are limited, and there is constant debate about the best use of those funds. Should research on a vaccine against AIDS be a priority? So far, researchers have had no success. Or should most of the resources be directed toward prevention? Or treatment? All of these are important. The problem is to determine where the available funds will provide the most benefit and to balance the very real suffering of people now living with AIDS with developing a long-term solution that might diminish future suffering.

The second set of questions concerns how much international funding should be directed toward AIDS-related issues versus other diseases. Malaria, for example, is still rampant in sub-Saharan Africa, while drug-resistant strains of already widespread tuberculosis are becoming more prevalent worldwide. And basic health problems such as dysentery continue to be major cause of death for young children. How can we decide where to focus funds and efforts in a way that is fair to all those who suffer the effects of health-related problems around the world?

CHRISTIAN RESPONSES

Christian responses to AIDS have varied from moralistic to supportive. In the early days when AIDS was first identified, churches frequently treated AIDS as punishment from God. Those who contracted the disease were often shunned or attacked, and a common assumption both in Africa and North America was that those suffering from AIDS had brought the disease on themselves through immoral behavior.

This attitude is destructive and unworthy of followers of Christ. First, it is factually incorrect: many people who are HIV positive have not engaged in risky or immoral behavior. Worse, it brings dishonor on the community of faith called to live out God's love and concern for people who are sick and suffering. The gospels do not restrict the call for Christians to love only those who are without sin—we are called to love *especially* those who are sick, imprisoned, and desperate.

Although the response from churches in the early days of the AIDS crisis has not always lived up to this high calling, and although some churches continue to treat AIDS as a reason for exclusion, most denominations have responded to the AIDS crisis with a wholehearted attempt to live out the demands of the gospel. The Christian Reformed World Relief Committee, for example, has developed a program called "Embrace AIDS" that integrates care for individuals living with AIDS, support and education services for families and communities, and partnerships with local churches to ensure that these programs are effective and sustainable. Such programs are more the norm than the exception in the larger denominations. In addition some evangelical nondenominational churches have mobilized their members to respond to AIDS. In 2007, Saddleback Church in California hosted the Global Summit on AIDS and the Church. Their website offers information and resources for Christians to connect with others in the fight against AIDS, malaria, and tuberculosis.

> "If you could only work with people you agree with, you will rule out the entire world."
>
> —Rick Warren, pastor of Saddleback Church, sharing strategies for addressing HIV/AIDS

With respect to government and World Health Organization responses to AIDS, North American evangelicals have not spoken with a unified voice. In June 2006 *Christianity Today* reported that a number of prominent evangelical leaders opposed United States aid dollars going to support the Global Fund to Fight AIDS, Tuberculosis, and Malaria. James Dobson, leader of Focus on the Family, criticized the Senate's vote to increase funding for the Global Fund, arguing that the membership of its board of directors, its spending decisions, and its promotion of condom use in preference to abstinence made it an unacceptable organization. In response, other prominent evangelical leaders, including Tony Campolo, argued that the problematic spending made up only a minute part of its total budget, while the Fund supported the work of numerous Christian organizations, including World Vision and the Salvation Army. Given the prominence of individuals on both sides of this debate, it is likely that Christian communities will continue to disagree about funding issues.

Although Christians are likely to disagree, it is imperative that we conduct those disagreements in a spirit of charity and forbearance. And we must not allow our disagreements to distract our attention from the important issues of our day. The world needs Christians to respond to the HIV/AIDS crisis in productive and loving ways. And the need is sufficiently great that every church can contribute in some way or another, whether through providing support and education, as many African churches do, or providing funding and medical supplies, as many Western churches do. We won't see the end of health problems in the world until God's kingdom has fully come, but in the meantime we can be imitators of Christ, offering healing and love to the world's needy.

Questions for Reflection and Discussion

1. Given limited funds, should public health officials focus on prevention of the spread of HIV or treatment of those already infected by HIV? How should these two be balanced?

2. When Christians disagree about issues like advocating the use of condoms as part of an AIDS prevention strategy, their disagreements sometimes get in the way of a productive response. In what ways can Christians who disagree about particulars still come together to address the global HIV/AIDS crisis?

3. The story at the beginning of the chapter raises issues of confidentiality and economics with respect to AIDS. Should council members at Covenant Redeemer Church be open about the family's HIV status, or should they keep that information confidential? Why? And if they cannot get health care treatment through Medicare, does the church have the responsibility to pay? Why?

For Further Reading

Cimperman, Maria. *When God's People Have HIV/AIDS: An Approach to Ethics.* Maryknoll, N.Y.: Orbis Books, 2005.

Keenan, James F., ed., with Jon D. Fuller, Lisa Sowle Cahill, and Kevin Kelly. *Catholic Ethicists on HIV/AIDS Prevention.* New York: Continuum, 2000.

Yamamori, Tesunao. *The Hope Factor: Engaging the Church in the HIV/AIDS Crisis.* Waynesboro, Ga.: Authentic Media, 2003.

CHAPTER 11

CONCLUDING THOUGHTS

"T hen the angel showed me the river of the water of life, as clear as crystal, flowing from the throne of God and of the Lamb down the middle of the great street of the city. On each side of the river stood the tree of life, bearing twelve crops of fruit, yielding its fruit every month. And the leaves of the tree are for the healing of the nations."

—Revelation 22:1-2

Health and life are two of the greatest gifts God has given us. When we can extend these gifts to others around us we mirror, in a small way, the activity and the intention of our gracious God. Health care is a human activity that brings small glimpses of the heavenly city into the contemporary world, and it is meant for all the nations, not just the rich and powerful ones.

Medicine can do wonderful things to heal us and to extend our lives. But the effects of sin are evident when we begin to worship modern technology and its ability to extend life at any cost and when we make an idol of health and life, putting our trust in them instead of the true God. And as long as the benefits of medicine go only to the rich while the poor continue to live in misery and deprivation, the injustice cries out for a compassionate response.

The story of Scripture offers Christians a powerful set of principles for understanding how good gifts like health and medicine can be misused or abused. We know that this is God's good world; that God's will for us is to enjoy life and health. We also know that all of God's good gifts become corrupted when we misuse them—and inevitably we do misuse them. We face the challenge of participating in God's redemption of the broken and sinful structures of this world, of doing what we can to rectify injustice and avoid idolatry. Above all, we recognize that true and full redemption comes only with God's final recreation of the world.

Thinking about bioethics as Christians, then, allows us to see the goodness of modern medicine without losing sight of the many ways it can be misused. In this book we've tried to maintain this balance—to celebrate the way transplant technology, for example, can give new life to someone condemned to death. At the same time, we also recognize the many ways that medicine tempts us to worship technology and science rather than the God who made them possible. And we see the sinful structures of a world where some people's medical needs are met without regard to cost and others die for lack of the most basic and inexpensive health care.

We also know that we are called to care for our neighbors, and that these neighbors are not limited to the members of our immediate families or our churches or even our fellow citizens. When Jesus told us to love even our enemies, he called us to the daunting task of trying to show love to all, and especially to those who are hungry, sick, or outcast from society. The tree of life is for the healing of all the nations, not just the wealthy, developed ones.

Modern medicine is a large, complex system, and none of us is in a position to radically change the way health care is delivered. But that does not excuse us from our responsibility to think carefully about what is right and what is problematic about health care in the contemporary world, why these problems arise, and what possible solutions are available. Further, we need to understand what responses to ethical issues have worked well in the past and which have not worked well. Uninformed reactions to perceived problems are likely to generate new problems while doing little to fix the original one; the more we understand the complexities of a situation, the better we can respond to it.

Over the course of this book we've looked at a number of specific structural issues that have arisen over and over again, both at the personal level and at the national and international levels. Consider, for example, assisted reproduction. Modern technology can offer techniques to infertile couples that can be a real blessing to them. At the same time, the availability of reproductive technologies tempts us to pursue them at all costs, sometimes to the point of idolatry, sometimes at the expense of risky techniques that may harm the child the couple hopes to conceive. For those in the midst of treatment, it is difficult to maintain perspective—every feature of the treatment focuses attention on possible success, and it's easy to lose sight of other concerns that should balance the pursuit of reproduction.

As individuals, we are rarely in a position to recognize the point past which a worthy goal becomes inappropriate. But in the context of a Christian community that helps us maintain perspective, that supports us and cautions us and loves us, we have a far better chance of using assisted reproductive technologies appropriately. God did not create us to live as isolated individuals. We reason better when we reason together, and we live better when we are members of a community that holds us accountable for our decisions.

This is equally true of decision-making at the state, national, and international levels. As a nation, we need to include the voices of all members of the community in our decisions about how health care will be delivered and who will have access to what treatments. The hard work of reaching democratic agreement on these issues can't be avoided if we hope to create a fair and equitable system.

If we fail to work toward a system that generates consensus, we are likely to end up doing injustice to large numbers of our fellow citizens. Those of us who are fortunate enough to have insurance and access to decent health care may find it easy to forget the poor while focusing on our own wants and needs. But as the Scriptures remind us, God always hears the cries of the poor and distressed. And this is even truer when we think about the world's needs and the imbalance of health care between developed and developing nations. If we fail to listen to the voices of our fellow Christians in Tanzania, Ghana, Brazil, the Philippines, and around the world, God will hold us accountable.

How can we as Christians make our impact felt? First, as we noted in the introduction, an adequate bioethics requires us to situate bioethical questions in community. Local communities are the best place for thinking about individual treatment decisions; broader communities are needed for thinking about adequate health care at the national and international levels. At every level, though, Christians need to provide an alternative to the individualism of contemporary health care.

Second, we need to recognize the ways health care structures can take on a life of their own. In chapter 1 we used the biblical language of "powers" to analyze social structures. These powers are not intrinsically evil. As part of God's creation and as essential aspects of human life they can do many good things, and we cannot live without them. But they are powers, and power magnifies corruption. For example, Western capitalism enables economic growth and vitality, but it can also oppress the poor and make access to adequate health care impossible for many. Unless we learn to step back and keep health care technology in perspective, we can get swept up in the power of medicine and fail to see its troublesome aspects. Wisdom requires us to maintain a critical distance from the powers of this world, and to call them to account when they claim more than their due.

Third, as Christians considering a wide variety of health care issues, we need to make sure our approach is compatible with our calling. If we are called to be honest and loving, then we need to advocate for health care practices that encourage honesty and love. We can't practice the virtues of gentleness and compassion in the context of structures that force us to live as self-interested individuals. In the health care context, remembering our calling can help us think through the ways we debate health care practices. Bioethics gives rise to some of the most contentious contemporary moral issues today—including euthanasia and abortion—and we will certainly find ourselves debating them for years to come. But our disagreements need to be kept within the boundaries of Christian behavior, and our arguments need to be characterized by love, not acrimony and unfair attacks. Christ needs to be visible in everything we do, even in our fervent disagreements with others.

Finally, however, we need to recognize that the ultimate fulfillment of God's kingdom will not come as a result of our efforts. We live in a world where sin and evil infest every human structure. So it is better that we take small steps toward a solution rather than fail to make any change because we insist on solving the whole problem forever. This is particularly important to remember in the context of the hugely complex issues of world poverty and the global spread of HIV/AIDS. These problems can seem so overwhelming that we simply give up and do nothing. As Jesus reminds us in the parable of the talents (Matt. 25:14-30), we must do what we can with what we have. We won't be held accountable for trying to use whatever resources we have available to respond to these issues—but we will be judged if we keep what little we have for ourselves.

BIBLIOGRAPHY

American Diabetes Association. "Economic Costs of Diabetes in the U.S. in 2007." *Diabetes Care* 31: 596-615, 2008.

Anspach, Renée R. *Deciding Who Lives: Fateful Choices in the Intensive-Care Nursery.* Berkeley: University of California Press, 1997.

Bate, Stuart C. "Counseling: Difference in Confessional Advice in South Africa." *Catholic Ethicists on HIV/AIDS Prevention*, James F. Keenan, Jon D. Fuller, Lisa Sowle Cahill, and Kevin Kelly, eds. New York: Continuum, 2000.

BBC. "Plugging the Brain Drain," 2005. http://news.bbc.co.uk/2/hi/africa/4339947.stm.

Bongmba, Elias K. *Facing a Pandemic: The African Church and the Crisis of HIV/AIDS.* Waco: Baylor University Press, 2007.

Burke, Daniel. "Rift Opens Among Evangelicals on AIDS Funding." *Christianity Today*, June 2006. http://www.christianitytoday.com/ct/2006/juneweb-only/122-52.0.html.

Cahill, Lisa Sowle. *Theological Bioethics: Participation, Justice, and Change.* Washington, D.C.: Georgetown University Press, 2005.

Campbell, Alastair V. *Health as Liberation: Medicine, Theology, and the Quest for Justice.* Cleveland: Pilgrim Press, 1995.

Caplan, Arthur. *Am I My Brother's Keeper? The Ethical Frontiers of Bio-medicine.* Bloomington: Indiana University Press, 1997.

Capron, Alexander Morgan. "In re Helga Wanglie." *Hastings Center Report,* 1991. 21(5): 26-28.

Cassell, Eric J. *Doctoring: The Nature of Primary Care Medicine*, New York: Oxford University Press, 1997.

Chalmers Center. "Doing Short-Term Missions without Doing Long-Term Harm." http://www.chalmers.org/staging/mandate/april_2008/stm.php. 2008.

Chambliss, Linda R. "Domestic Violence: A Public Health Crisis." *Clinical Obstetrics and Gynecology,* 1997. 40(3): 630-638.

Christian Reformed World Relief Committee (CRWRC). http://www.crcna.org/pages/crwrc_aids.cfm.

Colson, Charles. "Can We Prevent the 'Abolition of Man'? C.S. Lewis's Challenge to the Twenty-first Century." *Human Dignity in the Bio-tech Century: A Christian Vision for Public Policy*, Charles Colson and Nigel M. de S. Cameron, eds. Downers Grove, Ill.: InterVarsity Press, 2004. pp 11-20.

Condit, Celeste Michelle. *Decoding Abortion Rhetoric: Communicating Social Change.* Urbana: University of Illinois Press, 1990.

Evans, Abigail Rian. *Redeeming Marketplace Medicine: A Theology of Health Care.* Cleveland: Pilgrim Press, 1999.

Feder, Jody. "State Laws on Human Cloning." Washington, D.C.: Congressional Research Service, Library of Congress, 2003. http://www.usembassy.at/en/download/pdf/human_clone.pdf.

Fuller, Jon D. and James F. Keenan. "Introduction: At the End of the First Generation of HIV Prevention." *Catholic Ethicists on HIV/AIDS Prevention*, James F. Keenan, Jon D. Fuller, Lisa Sowle Cahill, and Kevin Kelly, eds. New York: Continuum, 2000. pp. 21-27.

Halevy, Amir, & Baruch Brody. "Brain Death: Reconciling Definitions, Criteria, and Tests." *Annals of Internal Medicine,* 1993. 119(6): 519-525.

Harrison, Beverly Wildung. *Making the Connections: Essays in Feminist Social Ethics.* Boston: Beacon Press, 1985.

Hui. Edwin C. *At the Beginning of Life: Dilemmas in Theological Bioethics.* Downer's Grove, Ill.: InterVarsity Press, 2002.

Iliffe, John. *The African AIDS Epidemic: A History.* Athens: Ohio University Press, 2006.

Kilner, John F., Nigel M. de S. Cameron, and David Schiedermayer. *Bioethics and the Future of Medicine: A Christian Appraisal.* Grand Rapids, Mich.: Eerdmans, 1995.

Knowles, Lori P. "The Governance of Reprogenetic Technology: International Models." *Reprogenetics: Law, Policy, and Ethical Issues*, Lori P. Knowles and Gregory E. Kaebnick, eds. Baltimore: The Johns Hopkins University Press, 2007. pp. 127-143.

Maguire, Daniel. *Sacred Choices: The Right to Contraception and Abortion in Ten World Religions.* Minneapolis: Augsburg Fortress Press, 2001

May, William F. *The Patient's Ordeal.* Bloomington: Indiana University Press, 1991.

Meilaender, Gilbert. *Bioethics: A Primer for Christians.* Grand Rapids: Mich.: Eerdmans. 1996.

Mitchell, C. Ben, Edmund Pellegrino, Jean Bethke Elshtain, John F. Kilner, and Scott B. Rae. *Bioetchnology and the Human Good.* Washington, D.C.: Georgetown University Press, 2007.

Mohrmann, Margaret E. *Medicine as Ministry: Reflections on Suffering, Ethics and Hope.* Cleveland: Pilgrim Press, 1995.

National Institutes of Health (NIH). http://www.nih.gov/.

O'Neil, Edward Jr. *Awakening Hippocrates: A Primer on Health, Poverty, and Global Service.* Chicago: American Medical Association Press, 2006.

Outka, Gene. "The Ethics of Human Stem Cell Research." *God and the Embryo: Religious Voices on Cloning and Stem Cell Research*, Brent Waters and Ronald Cole-Turner, eds. Washington, D.C.: Georgetown University Press, 2003. pp. 29-64.

Pence, Gregory E. *Medical Ethics: Accounts of the Cases that Shaped and Define Medical Ethics 5ᵗʰ Ed.* New York: McGraw-Hill, 2008.

Peters, Ted and Gaymon Bennett. "A Plea for Beneficence." *God and the Embryo: Religious Voices on Cloning and Stem Cell Research*, Brent Waters and Ronald Cole-Turner, eds. Washington, D.C.: Georgetown University Press, 2003. pp. 111-130.

Peters, Ted. "Embryonic Stem Cells and the Theology of Dignity." *The Human Embryonic Stem Cell Debate: Science, Ethics and Public Policy*, Suzanne Holland, Karen Lebacqz and Laurie Zoloth, eds. Cambridge, Mass.: The MIT Press, 2001. pp. 127-139.

Phillips, Susan P. "Violence and abortions: What's a doctor to do?" *CMAJ*, 2005. 172 (5): 653.

President's Council on Bioethics. *Human Cloning and Human Dignity: The Report of the President's Council on Bioethics.* New York: Public Affairs, 2002.

Riverson, Joe W. deGraft Johnson. "Water Sustains Life and Health." *Transforming Health: Christian Approaches to Healing and Wholeness*, Eric Ram, ed. Monrovia, Calif.: MARC Publications, 1995. pp. 137-154.

Rothman, Barbara Katz. *Recreating Motherhood: Ideology and Technology in a Patriarchal Society.* New York: W.W. Norton & Company, 1989.

Rudy, Kathy. *Beyond Pro-Life and Pro-Choice: Moral Diversity in the Abortion Debate.* Boston: Beacon Press, 1996.

Ryan, Maura. *Ethics and Economics of Assisted Reproduction: The Cost of Longing.* Washington, D.C.: Georgetown University Press, 2001.

Sachs, Jeffrey. *The End of Poverty: Economic Possibilities for Our Time.* New York: Penguin Press, 2005.

Shuman, Joel James and Brian Volck. *Reclaiming the Body: Christians and the Faithful Use of Modern Medicine.* Grand Rapids, Mich.: Brazos Press, 2006.

Shuman, Joel James and Keith Meador. *Heal Thyself: Spirituality, Medicine, and the Distortion of Christianity.* Oxford: Oxford University Press, 2003.

Smith, H. W. and Cindy Kronauge. "The Politics of Abortion: Husband Notification Legislation, Self-Disclosure, and Marital Bargaining." *The Sociological Quarterly,* 1990. 31(4): 585-598.

Suchdev, Parminder, Kym Ahrens, Eleanor Click, Lori Macklin, Doris Evangelista and Elinor Graham. "A Model for Sustainable Short-Term International Medical Trips." *Ambulatory Pediatrics,* 2007. Vol. 7, no. 4: 317-320.

Thomson, Judith Jarvis. *Rights, Restitution, and Risk: Essays in Moral Theory.* Cambridge, Mass.: Harvard University Press, 1986.

Toombs, S. Kay, David Barnard and Ronald A. Carson, eds. *Chronic Illness: From Experience to Policy.* Bloomington: Indiana University Press, 1995.

Van Leeuwen, Mary Stewart. *My Brother's Keeper: What the Social Sciences Do (and Don't) Tell Us about Masculinity.* Downer's Grove, IL: Intervarsity Press, 2002.

Verhey, Allen. *Reading the Bible in the Strange World of Medicine,* Grand Rapids, Mich.: Eerdmans, 2003.

Waters, Brent. *Reproductive Technology: Towards a Theology of Procreative Stewardship.* Cleveland: Pilgrim Press, 2001.

World Health Organization. *World Health Statistics.* Geneva, WHO Press, 2008. Available at http://www.who.int/en/.

Zoloth, Laurie. "Freedoms, Duties, and Limits: The Ethics of Research in Human Stem Cells." *God and the Embryo: Religious Voices on Stem Cells and Cloning,* Brent Waters and Ronald Cole-Turner, eds. Washington, D.C.: Georgetown University Press, 2003. pp. 141-151.